ESSENTIAL CONCEPTS OF ELECTROPHYSIOLOGY AND PACING THROUGH CASE STUDIES

ESSENTIAL CONCEPTS OF ELECTROPHYSIOLOGY AND PACING THROUGH CASE STUDIES

EDITED BY

Kenneth A. Ellenbogen, MD

CONTRIBUTORS

Roderick Tung, MD

Prabal K. Guha, MD

Jeanine Leffler, RN

Kevin D. Oakeson, MS

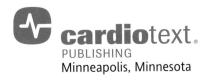

cardiotext

PUBLISHING

Minneapolis, Minnesota

© 2014 Kenneth A. Ellenbogen, Roderick Tung, Prabal K. Guha, Jeanine Leffler, Kevin D. Oakeson

Cardiotext Publishing, LLC
3405 W. 44th Street
Minneapolis, Minnesota 55410
USA

www.cardiotextpublishing.com

Any updates to this book may be found at:
www.cardiotextpublishing.com/essential-concepts-of-electrophysiology-and-pacing-through-case-studies

Comments, inquiries, and requests for bulk sales can be directed to the publisher at: info@cardiotextpublishing.com.

Library of Congress Control Number: 2013954649

ISBN: 978-1-935395-85-0

eISBN: 978-1-935395-99-7

Printed in the United States of America

Dedication

To Mark E. Josephson, MD, our friend and mentor whose life and work has been a constant source of inspiration and encouragement and who continues to challenge us to advance the science of arrhythmias.

In memory of Mark A. Wood, MD, my friend and colleague whose life will always be remembered.

—Kenneth A. Ellenbogen, MD

Contents

About the Contributors

Editor:

Kenneth A. Ellenbogen, MD, FACC, is Director of Clinical Cardiac Electrophysiology and Pacing, Chair of the Division of Cardiology at the Pauley Heart Center, and Kontos Endowed Professor at Virginia Commonwealth University's Medical College of Virginia, Richmond, Virginia.

Contributors:

Roderick Tung, MD, FACC, FHRS, is Assistant Professor of Medicine and Director of the Specialized Program for Ventricular Tachycardia at the UCLA Cardiac Arrhythmia Center, UCLA Ronald Reagan Medical Center, Los Angeles, California.

Prabal K. Guha, MD, FACC, is Director of the Electrophysiology Laboratory at Carolinas Hospital, Florence, South Carolina.

Jeanine Leffler, RN, is a field clinical representative in Richmond, Virginia.

Kevin D. Oakeson, MS, is a clinical field engineer in Boston, Massachusetts.

Preface

One of the most essential skills in electrophysiology is the ability to analyze tracings. The scope of our practice has changed dramatically, and the tracings can range from the surface electrocardiogram, to pacemaker/ICD recordings, and finally, to complex intracardiac tracings. We have tried to cover a sampling of tracings that cover the range of these experiences with a collection of basic, intermediate and challenging cases from all these areas. By doing this, we have created a volume that is useful to electrophysiology technicians, electrophysiology and pacing nurses, pacemaker and ablation field representatives and engineers, and especially electrophysiology fellows and physicians.

Each case includes relevant references that allow the reader to review the initial description of a particular pacing maneuver or the concept illustrated by the tracing(s). We have tried to focus on some of the fundamental concepts that underlie electrophysiology and pacing to provide an opportunity to review these important lessons.

We have enjoyed selecting and annotating these cases, and we hope that this book will prove useful to students and professionals preparing for the wide range of examinations that cover these areas as well as an educational and challenging learning experience.

—Kenneth A. Ellenbogen, MD
Richmond, Virginia

Roderick Tung, MD
Los Angeles, California

Prabal K. Guha, MD
Florence, South Carolina

Jeanine Leffler, RN
Richmond, Virginia

Kevin D. Oakeson, MS
Boston, Massachusetts

Abbreviations

ABP	atrial blanking period		MTR	maximal tracking rate
ATP	antitachycardia pacing		MVP	managed ventricular pacing
AV	atrioventricular		NICM	nonischemic cardiomyopathy
AVNRT	atrioventricular nodal reentrant tachycardia		NSVT	nonsustained ventricular tachycardia
BBR	bundle branch reentry		PAC	premature atrial contraction
CHF	congestive heart failure		PMT	pacemaker-mediated tachycardia
CL	cycle length		PPI	postpacing interval
CS	coronary sinus		PV	pulmonary vein
DFT	defibrillation threshold		PVARP	postventricular atrial refractory period
ECG	electrocardiogram		PVC	premature ventricular contraction
EF	ejection fraction		RBBB	right bundle branch block
EGM	electrogram		RCC	right coronary cusp
EMI	electromagnetic interference		RV	right ventricle or right ventricular
FFRW	far-field R wave		SICD	subcutaneous implantable cardiac defibrillator
ICD	implantable cardiac defibrillator		SVT	supraventricular tachycardia
ILR	implantable loop recorder		TCL	tachycardia cycle length
JT	junctional tachycardia		VA	ventricular arrhythmia
LBBB	left bundle branch block		VF	ventricular fibrillation
LCC	left coronary cusp		VP	ventricular pacing
LRI	lower rate interval		VSP	ventricular safety pacing
LV	left ventricle or left ventricular		VT	ventricular tachycardia
MI	myocardial infarction			

PART 1

ECG

Question

Where is the site of origin of this PVC in a 72-year-old man presenting with palpitations?

A) Anterolateral papillary muscle

B) Left posterior fascicle

C) Epicardial crux

D) Posteromedial papillary muscle

Figure 1.A.1

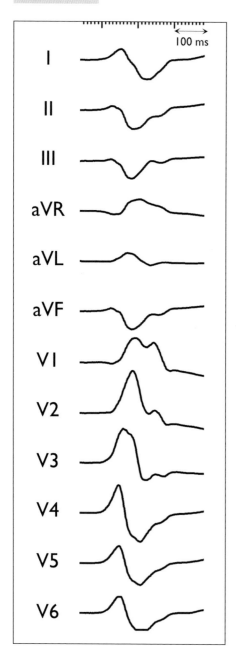

Figure 1.A.2

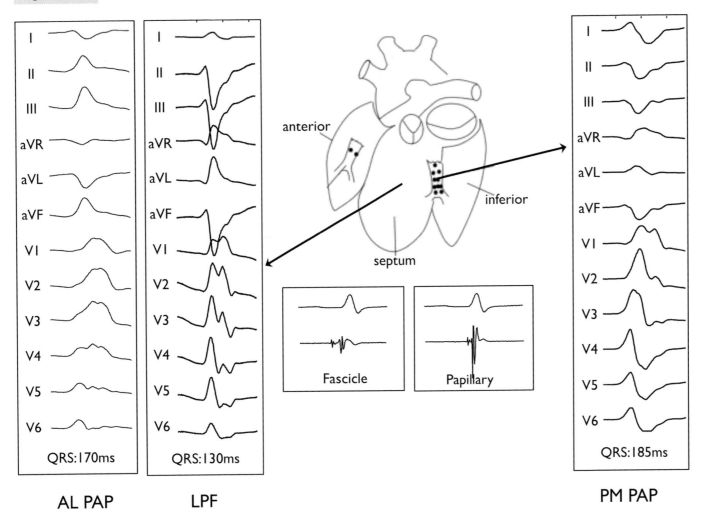

*A*nswer

The correct answer is **D**. This PVC originated from the **postero-medial papillary muscle** with history of infarction.

All of these sites of left ventricular origin have right bundle branch block left superior axis except the anterolateral papillary muscle, which has a right bundle branch block right inferior axis morphology. Crux of the heart sites of origin near the proximal CS have a characteristic sudden R wave from V_1 to V_2.

Differentiating posterior fascicular origin from posteromedial papillary muscle can be difficult. Due to proximity to the conduction system, left posterior fascicular QRS width is narrower (130 ms) than papillary muscle VT (185 ms), which has been shown to be the most reliable predictor. While ablation sites on papillary muscles may have Purkinje potentials (distal with later timing), the majority of fascicular target sites exhibit Purkinje potentials.

References

1. Yamada T, Doppalapudi H, McElderry HT, et al. Idiopathic ventricular arrhythmias originating from the papillary muscles in the left ventricle: prevalence, electrocardiographic and electrophysiologic characteristics, and results of the radiofrequency catheter ablation. *J Cardiovasc Electrophysiol.* 2010;21(1):62-69.
2. Good E, Good E, Desjardins B, et al. Ventricular arrhythmias originating from a papillary muscle in patients without prior infarction: a comparison with fascicular arrhythmias. *Heart Rhythm.* 2008;5(11):1530-1537.
3. Doppalapudi H, Yamada T, Ramasway K, Ahn J, Kay GN. Idiopathic focal epicardial ventricular tachycardia origination from the crux of the heart. *Heart Rhythm.* 2009;6(1):44-50.

Case 1.B

Question

What is the mechanism of this arrhythmia in an asymptomatic 65-year-old man?

A) Blocked premature atrial contractions

B) Concealed His extrasystoles

C) Sinus arrhythmia

D) Sinoatrial Wenckebach

Figure 1.B.1

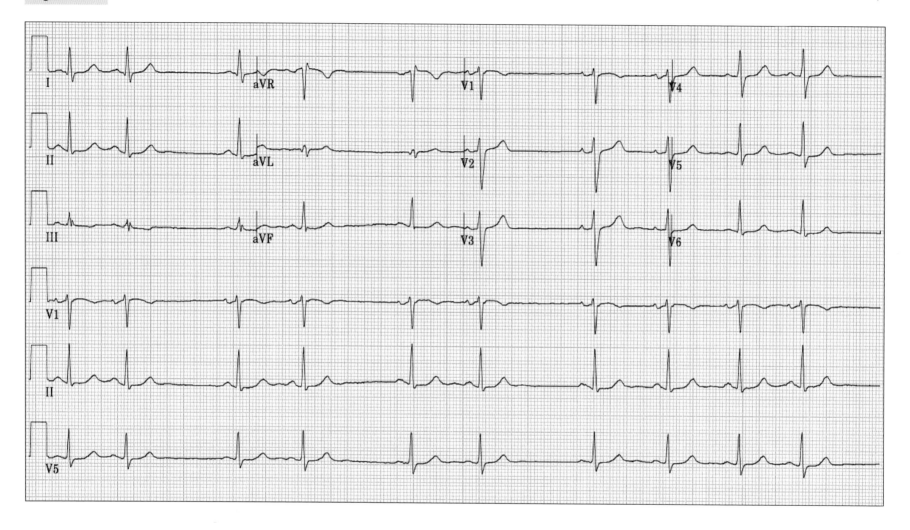

Figure 1.B.2

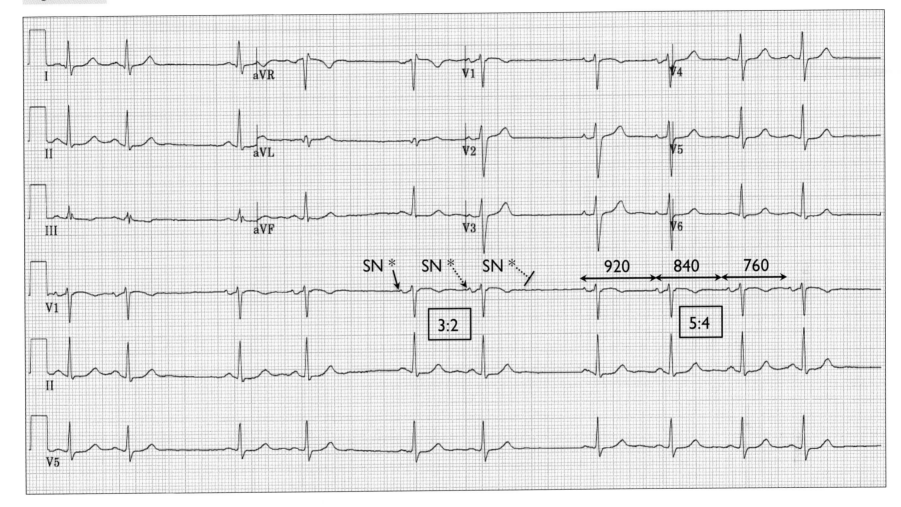

Answer

The correct answer is **D**. This tracing shows **sinoatrial Wenckebach**.

The periodicity is not suggestive of sinus arrhythmia, and dropped beats are not preceded by P waves, which excludes blocked premature atrial contractions. Concealed His extrasystoles should not result in sinus suppression in the absence of retrograde atrial conduction. Wenckebach phenomenon is defined as decremental conduction from a fixed source prior to block. Sinus node activity cannot be seen on the 12-lead ECG, and therefore conduction can only be inferred from the P-wave timing. First-degree conduction delay cannot be seen on surface ECG, and third-degree sinoatrial block is complete absence of the P wave.

Grouped beating should always suggest Wenckebach periodicity. The dropped P wave is not 2× the normal sinus cycle length, which is diagnostic of Mobitz II SA block. With a higher ratio of conducted sinus to P waves seen during 5:4, the PP intervals progressively shorten because the first decrement is longest in Wenckebach, which is comparable to progressive RR shortening in AV nodal Wenckebach.

References

1. Rothfeld EL, Bernstein A. Wenckebach block of sinoatrial conduction.
    Dis Chest. 1961;40:106.

2. Shamroth L, Dove E. The Wenckebach phenomenon in sino-atrial block.
    Br Heart J. 1966;28(3):350-358.

Question

Which of the following is the most likely site of origin for this ectopic beat in a 21-year-old man with palpitations?

A) Right ventricular outflow tract

B) Right/left coronary cusp junction

C) Noncoronary cusp

D) Aorto-mitral continuity

E) Left ventricular summit

Figure 1.C.1

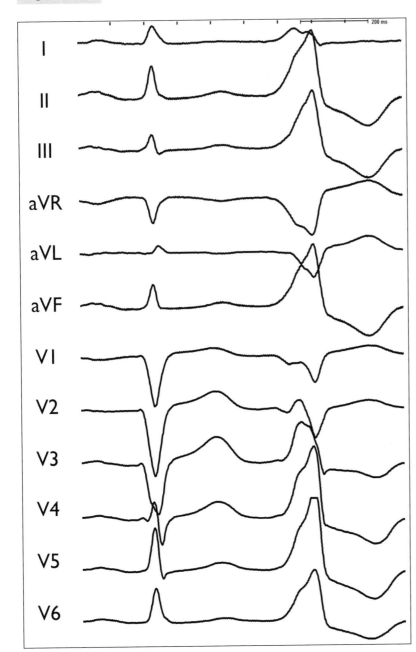

*A*nswer

The correct answer is **B**. This PVC suggests an origin at the **RCC/ LCC junction**.

The noncoronary cusp is predominantly atrial tissue and rarely is a site of origin for ventricular arrhythmias. Aorto-mitral continuity PVCs typically have a qR pattern in V_1, while a left ventricular summit origin has a dominant R-wave precordium with negative lead 1 and aVL. Right ventricular outflow tract origins typically have late precordial transitions after V_3.

Unique electrocardiographic features of the RCC/LCC junction have been described:

1. A notch in the downstroke of qS in V_1.

2. A transition at or before V_3 suggests left outflow tract over right outflow tract.

3. A qRS pattern in V_1–V_3 (seen in V_2). Outflow tract PVCs have a QS morphology in aVR and aVL.

Figure 1.C.2

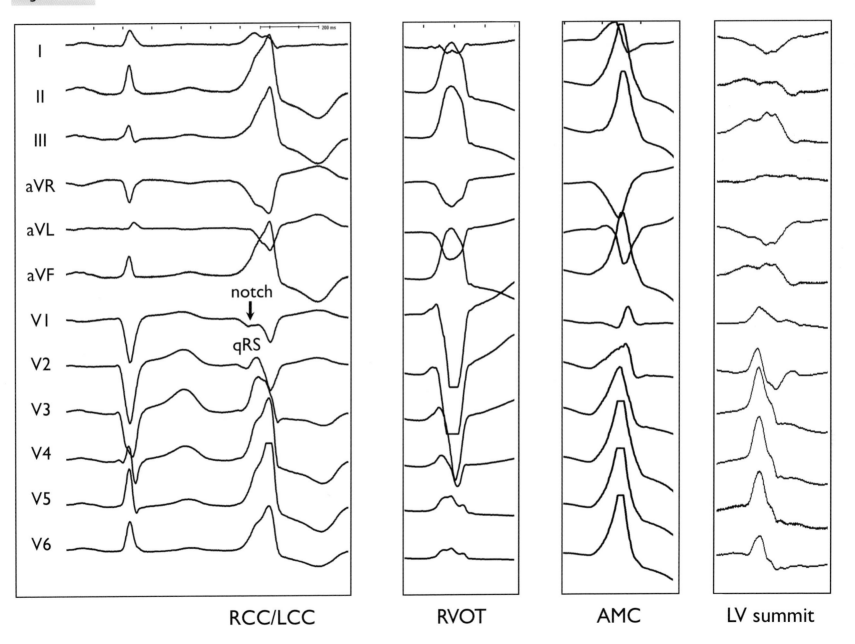

200 ms

I
II
III
aVR
aVL
aVF
V1
V2
V3
V4
V5
V6

notch

qRS

RCC/LCC   RVOT   AMC   LV summit

References

1.   Bala R, Garcia FC, Hutchinson MD, et al. Electrocardiographic and electrophysiologic features of ventricular arrhythmias originating from the right/left coronary cusp commissure. *Heart Rhythm*. 2010;7(3):312-322.

2.   Yamada T, Yoshida N, Murakami Y, et al. Electrocardiographic characteristics of ventricular arrhythmias originating from the junction of the left and right coronary sinuses of Valsalva in the aorta: the activation pattern as a rationale for electrocardiographic characteristics. *Heart Rhythm*. 2008;5(2):184-192.

Case **1.D**

Question

What is the most likely diagnosis in this 35-year-old woman with intermittent palpitations?

A) Blocked PACs

B) Wenckebach conduction

C) Concealed His extrasystoles

D) Typical AV nodal echo beats

Figure 1.D.1

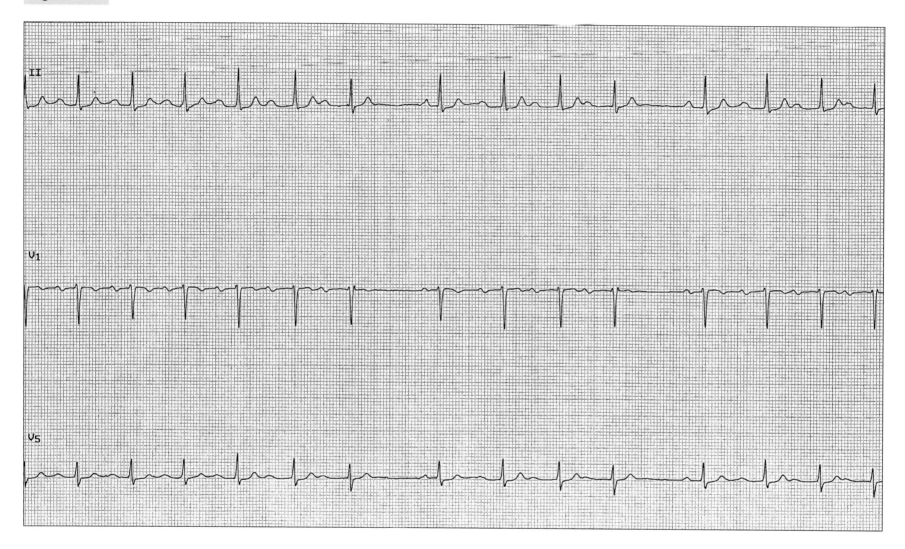

Figure 1.D.2

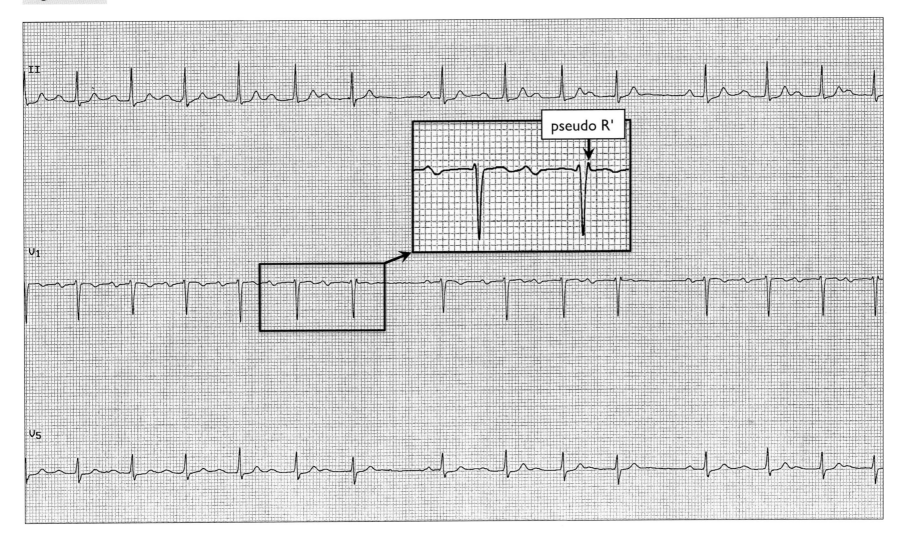

*A*nswer

The correct answer is **D**. Dual AV node physiology conduction is seen with a **typical slow–fast AV nodal echo.**

The differential diagnosis of grouped beating most frequently suggests Wenckebach conduction but can occur with blocked PACs or concealed His extrasystoles. True concealed extrasystoles are not seen on surface ECG, but usually account for unexplained delayed conduction. While PR prologation is seen, which represents a change in conduction down the slow pathway in sinus rhythm, the last atrial event prior to block is earlier than the expected sinus rhythm. Therefore, Wenckebach phenomenon is not present.

Rather, the last atrial event prior to block occurs at the end of the QRS, seen as a pseudo-R', which is highly suggestive of a typical AV nodal echo beat. An AV nodal echo beat resets the sinus node, resulting in a pause. The reproducible short, fixed coupling of this R' makes blocked PACs a less likely explanation.

Question

What is the first step in the management of this tracing?

A) Amiodarone

B) Magnesium

C) Overdrive pacing

D) No treatment

Figure 1.E.1

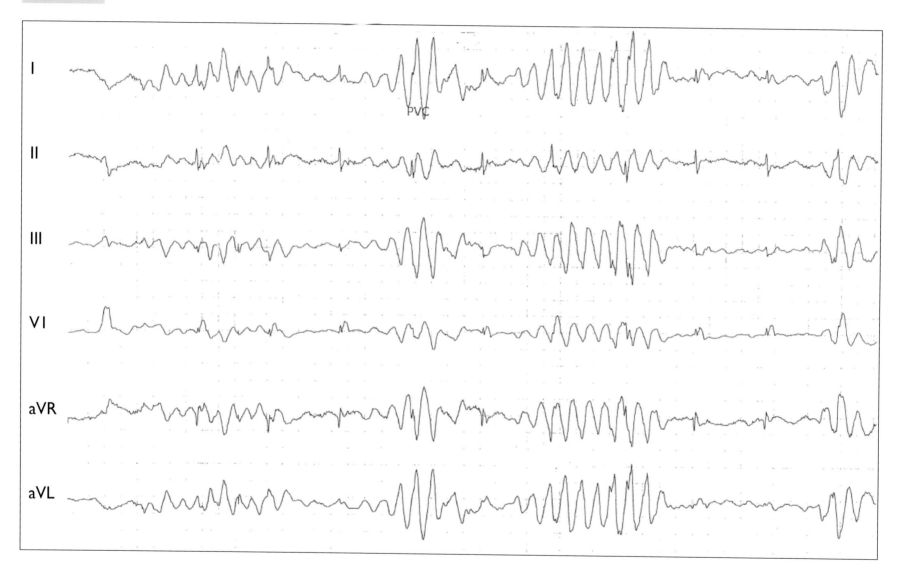

Figure 1.E.2

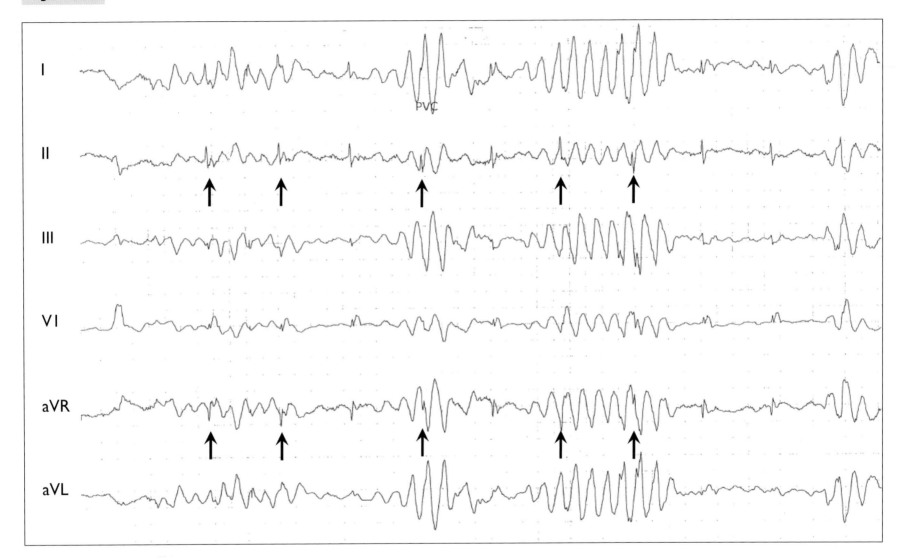

*A*nswer

The correct answer is **D. No treatment** is necessary, as this tracing exhibits artifact.

Baseline artifact is present, and the wide-complex beats that appear to be torsades de pointes are the result of physical movement and noise. QRS complexes are seen consistently throughout the strip, which makes it impossible for the wide complexes to represent ventricular depolarization.

Intravenous magnesium is the first therapy for torsades de pointes, and overdrive pacing can be helpful to eliminate pause-dependent initiations. Artifact is commonly seen in the inpatient setting on telemetry, and analysis of all leads is important for recognizing this phenomenon.

Reference

1. Knight B, Pelosi F, Michaud GF, Strickberger SA, Morady F. Clinical consequences of electrocardiographic artifact mimicking ventricular tachycardia. *N Engl J Med*. 1999;341(17):1270-1274.

Case 1.F

Question

What is the most likely substrate for ventricular tachycardia in this 69-year-old man?

A) Arrhythmogenic RV cardiomyopathy

B) Septal infarction

C) Anteroapical infarction

D) Nonischemic cardiomyopathy

Figure 1.F.1

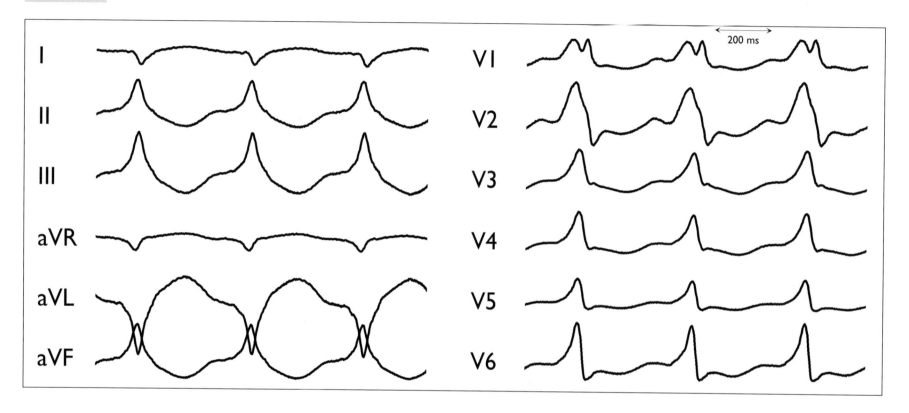

Figure 1.F.2

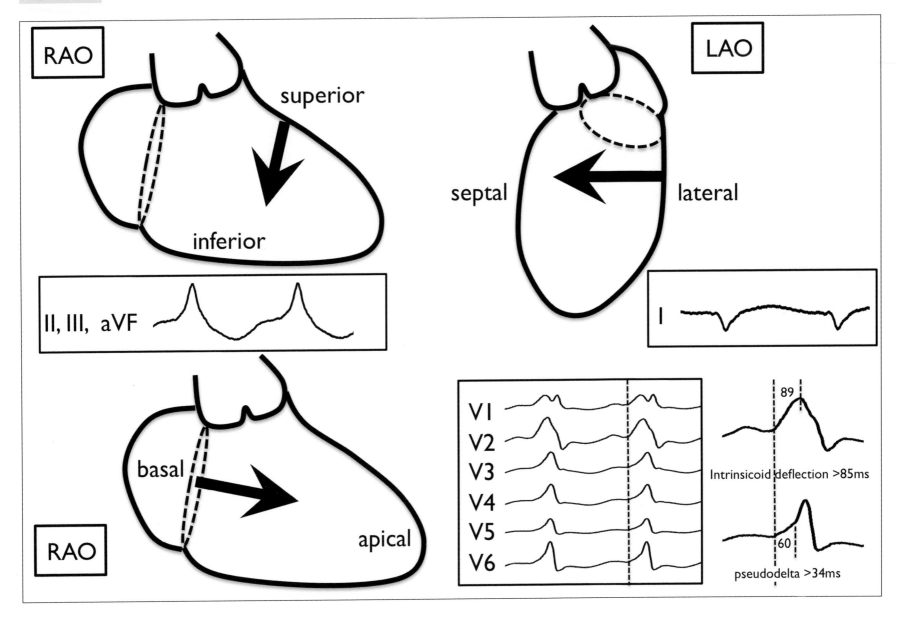

*A*nswer

The correct answer is **D**. This ventricular tachycardia (VT) from the basal anterolateral epicardium is most commonly seen in patients with **nonischemic cardiomyopathy** (NICM, idiopathic dilated).

Arrhythmogenic RV cardiomyopathy characteristically results in left bundle branch morphology VT. Patients with septal infarction may have left bundle or right bundle morphology VT. Lead I is typically positive with septal sites of origin and negative from the lateral free wall. This right bundle morphology has predominantly R waves across the precordium without a transition, suggesting a basal exit site. Apical sites exhibit negative precordial concordance with predominant qS complexes. The inferior leads help distinguish between inferior and superior sites.

NICM patients have scar in the basal perivalvular region of the left ventricle with a predilection for greater epicardial than endocardial fibrosis. In this case, the QRS is 190 ms and a delayed upstroke, or "slurring" (pseudo-delta >34 ms, intrinsicoid deflection >85 ms) is seen in the precordial leads suggesting an epicardial exit site morphology.

References

1. Josephson ME, Callans DJ. Using the twelve-lead electrocardiogram to localize the site of origin of ventricular tachycardia. *Heart Rhythm*. 2005;2(4):443-446.

2. Berruezo A, Mont L, Nava S, Cueca E, Bartholomay E, Brugada J. Electrocardiographic recognition of the epicardial origin of ventricular tachycardias. *Circulation*. 2004;109(15):1842-1847.

3. Cano O, Hutchinson M, Lin D, et al. Electroanatomic substrate and ablation outcome for suspected epicardial ventricular tachycardia in left ventricular nonischemic cardiomyopathy. *J Am Coll Cardiol*. 2009;54(9):799-808.

*Q*uestion

What is the most likely mechanism of arrhythmia in a 55-year-old man presenting to the emergency department with palpitations?

A) Supraventricular tachycardia with aberration

B) Antidromic reentry

C) Ventricular tachycardia

Figure 1.G.1

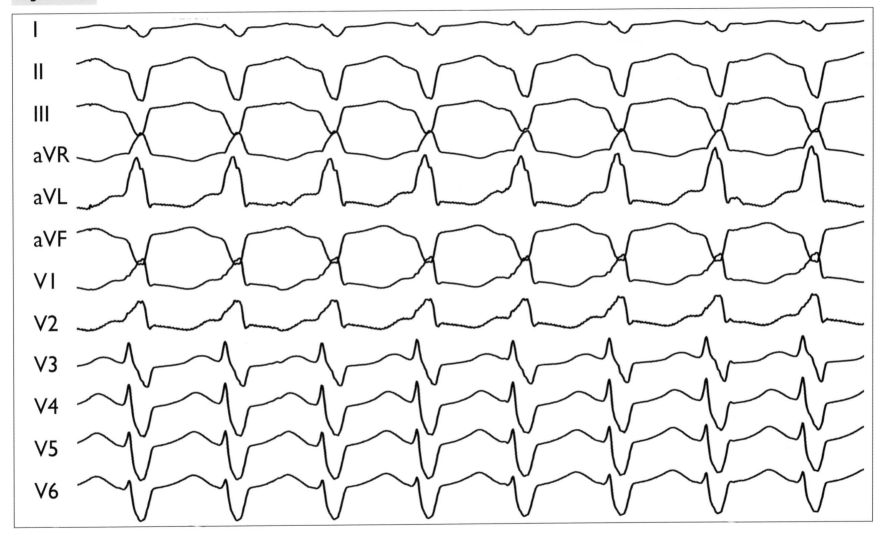

Figure 1.G.2

Classical, Wellens, criteria favoring VT	
AV dissociation, capture or fusion beats, negative or positive concordance, tachycardia QRS more narrow than sinus QRS	
RBBB configuration	LBBB configuration
QRS width >140 ms, left axis	QRS width >160 ms, right axis
QR, R, RSr' complex in V1 qR in V1 R in V1 Rabbit ear in V1	(A) Initial R in V1 >30 ms (B) Slurring or notching of the downstroke of the S wave in V1–2 (C) Begin QRS-nadir S wave >70 ms in V1–2
RS <1 in V6 QS in V6 	Any Q V6 Any Q in V6

Figure 1.G.3

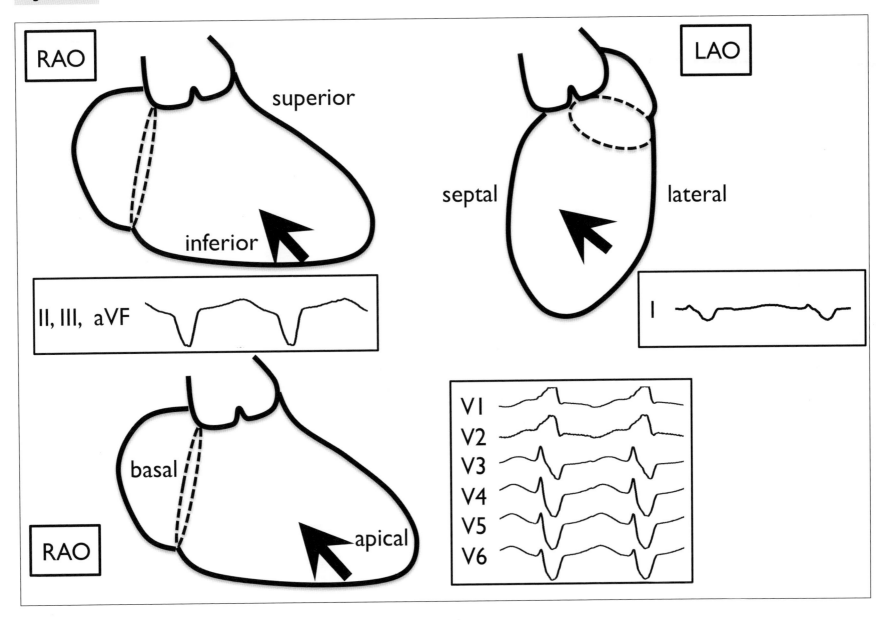

Answer

The correct answer is **C.** The wide-complex tachycardia is most consistent with **ventricular tachycardia (VT)** in a patient with inferior myocardial infarction.

Many features are useful for distinguishing supraventricular tachycardia with phase three aberration from VT. AV dissociation is specific for VT, although AV node reentry, concealed nodoventricular orthodromic tachycardia, and junctional tachycardia can all exhibit dissociated atrial activity. In this case, consistent P waves are not seen throughout the tracing. Fusion and capture beats, which are also highly suggestive of VT, are not seen.

A QRS width of >140 ms in right bundle morphology (>160 ms for LBBB) is specific for VT and, in this case, measures 150 ms. Importantly, the axis is northwest with positive initial R wave in aVR, suggesting activation toward the right shoulder from a more apical site of origin. This is supported by predominant S waves in the precordium starting at V_3. Lead I is net negative, suggesting exit from the lateral, rather than septal, side of the inferior scar. In a right bundle morphology, a monophasic R wave in V_1 and R/S ratio <1 in V_6 is supportive of VT. Antidromic tachycardia from a bypass tract typically has R wave–dominant precordium due to a basal annular ventricular insertion.

References

1. Vereckei A, Duray G, Szénási G, Altemose GT, Miller JM. New algorithm using only lead aVR for differential diagnosis of wide QRS complex tachycardia. *Heart Rhythm*. 2008;5(1):89-98.

2. Wellens HJ, Bar FW, Lie KI. The value of the electrocardiogram in the differential diagnosis of a tachycardia with a widened QRS complex. *Am J Med*. 1978;64:27-33.

3. Josephson ME, Callans DJ. Using the twelve-lead electrocardiogram to localize the site of origin of ventricular tachycardia. *Heart Rhythm*. 2005; 2(4):443-446.

Question

Where is the most likely site of this bypass tract?

A) Right free wall

B) Midseptal

C) Epicardial

D) Left lateral

Figure 1.H.1

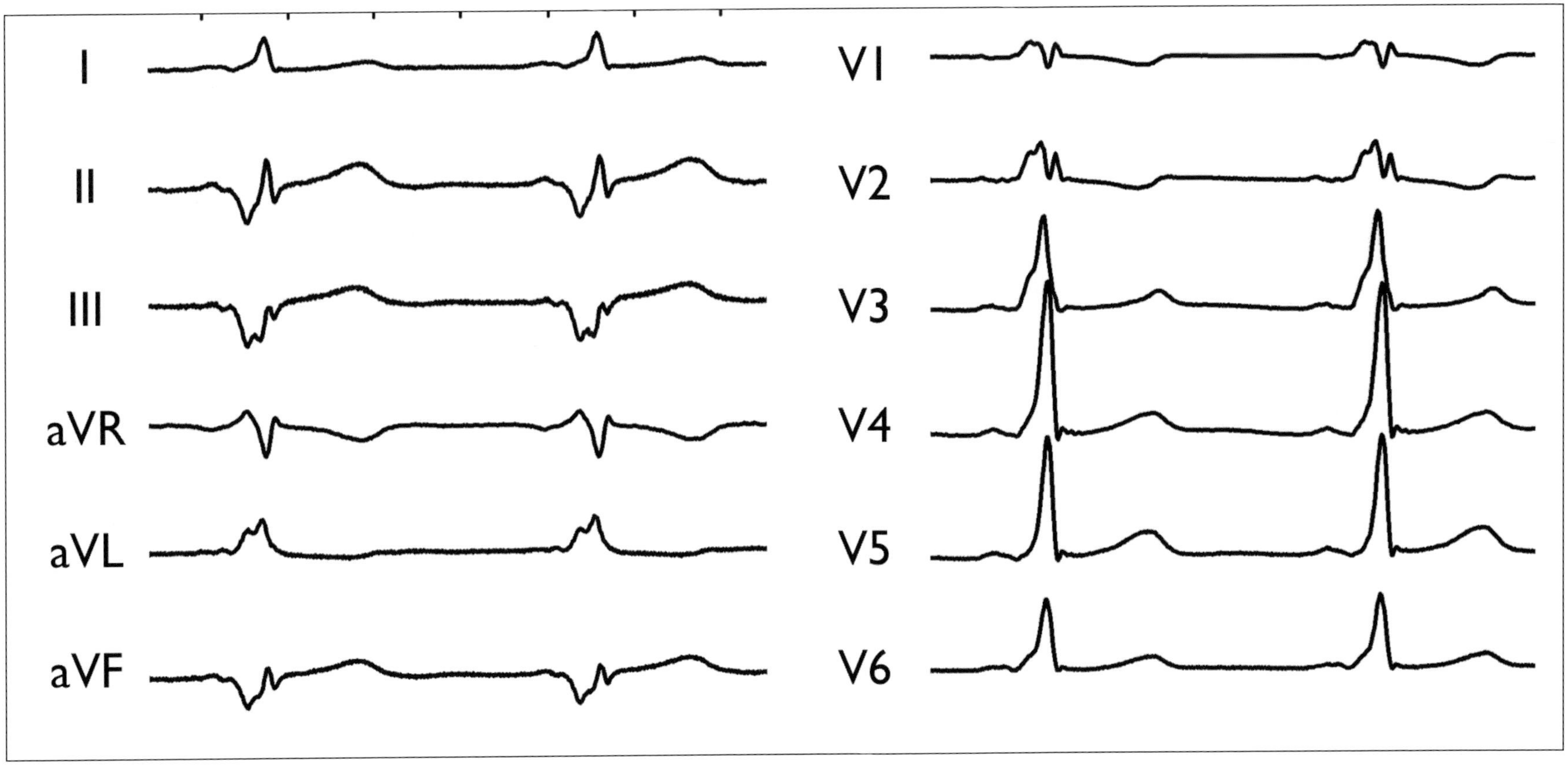

Figure 1.H.2

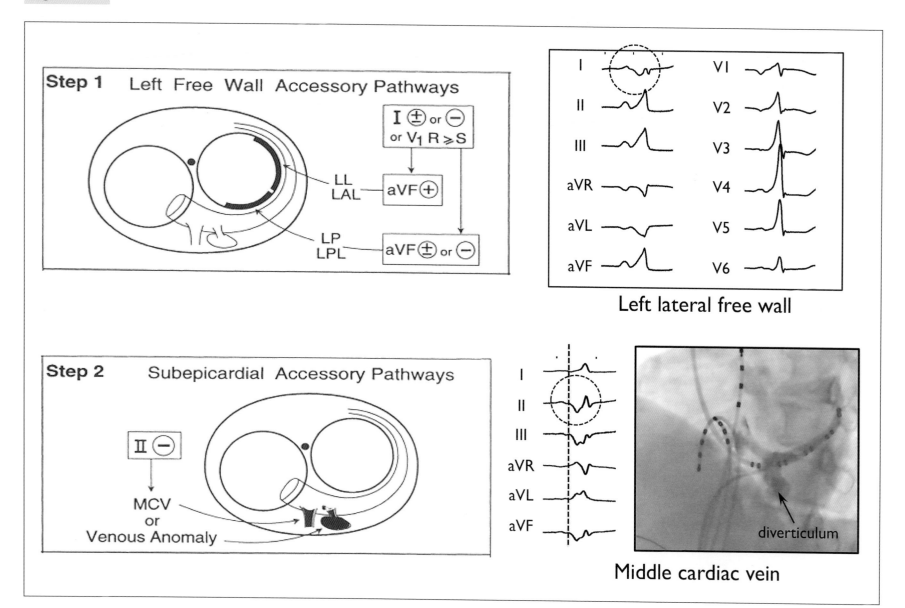

Left lateral free wall

Middle cardiac vein

Figure 1.H.3

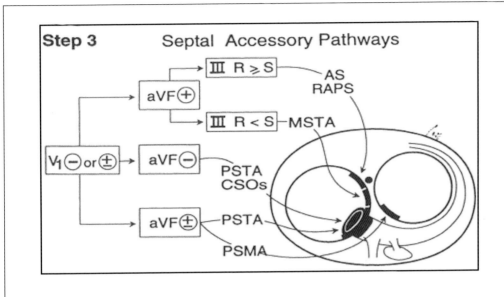

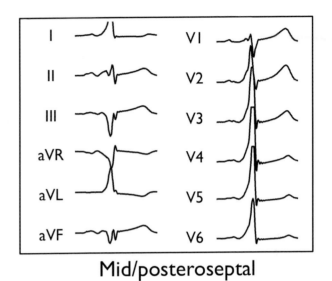

Mid/posteroseptal

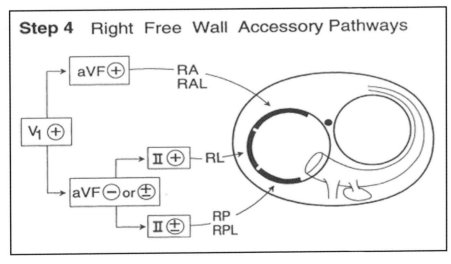

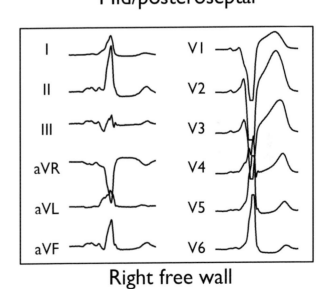

Right free wall

*A*nswer

The correct answer is **C**. The morphology is characteristic of an **epicardial** pathway location.

Many algorithms have been validated for localization of bypass tracts. A four-step algorithm by Arruda et al rapidly identifies left lateral wall pathways if the delta wave is isoelectric or negative in lead I. A QS pattern in lead II is specific for middle cardiac vein left posteroseptal pathway location. A diverticulum or pouch in the coronary sinus is often associated with this pattern.

Septal pathways may be on the right or left side of the septum and typically have isoelectric or negative delta wave in lead V_1. The absence of these characteristics leads to the diagnosis of a right free wall pathway. Additionally, the inscription of the delta wave prior to the completion of the P wave is highly suggestive of a right-sided pathway.

Reference

1. Arruda MS, McClelland JH, Wang X, et al. Development and validation of an ECG algorithm for identifying accessory pathway ablation
    site in Wolff-Parkinson-White syndrome. *J Cardiovasc Electrophysiol*.
    1998;9(1):2-12.

Question

What is the most likely diagnosis in this 65-year-old man presenting with palpitations?

A) Supraventricular tachycardia

B) Supraventricular tachycardia with aberration

C) Ventricular tachycardia

D) Pre-excited tachycardia (Mahaim)

Figure 1.I.1

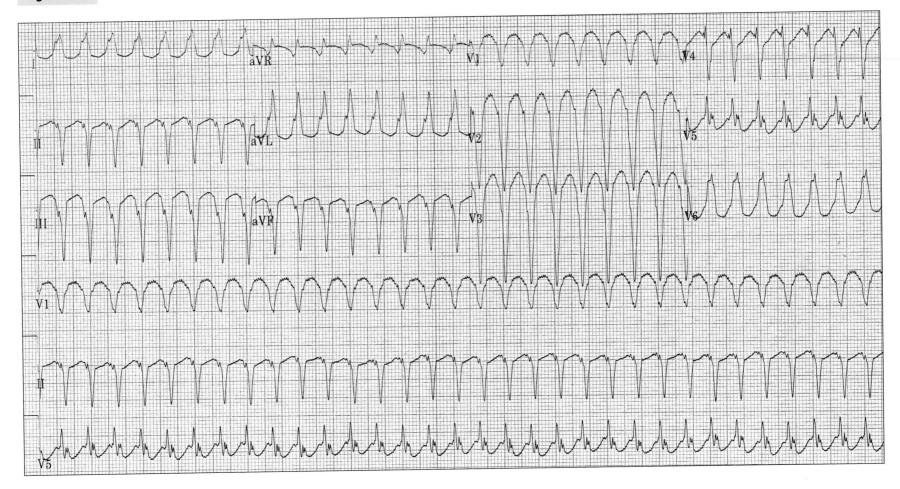

*A*nswer

The correct answer is **B**. This arrhythmia is most consistent with **supraventricular tachycardia (SVT) with aberration**.

The QRS width is 140 ms, and for left bundle branch morphology, a width of >160 ms supports the diagnosis of VT. Although an atriofascicular pathway does exhibit a left bundle branch block pattern with late transition, the QRS is typically wider in Mahaim tachycardia. The absence of an RS complex in the precordial leads and an R to S time of >100 ms in V_1 are also suggestive of VT by Brugada criteria. A Q wave in V_6 in the setting of a left bundle branch block morphology is highly suggestive of VT, although not present. In this case, the R to S time is 60 ms and a precordial transition consistent with a typical left bundle branch block is seen. AV dissociation is not evident in this tracing. The axis is leftward and the initial vector in aVR is negative, which is expected for a typical left bundle.

References

1. Wellens HJ, Bar FW, Lie KI. The value of the electrocardiogram in the differential diagnosis of a tachycardia with a widened QRS complex. *Am J Med.* 1978;64:27–33.

2. Brugada P, Brugada J, Mont L, Smeets J, Andries EW. A new approach to the differential diagnosis of a regular tachycardia with a wide QRS complex. *Circulation.* 1991;83(5):1649–1659.

3. Vereckei A, Duray G, Szénási G, Altemose GT, Miller JM. New algorithm using only lead aVR for differential diagnosis of wide QRS complex tachycardia. *Heart Rhythm.* 2008;5(1):89–98.

PART

2

Electrophysiology Concepts

Question

What does this entrainment response demonstrate?

A) Failure to capture

B) Pacing just outside of an isthmus

C) Concealed intracardiac fusion

D) Pacing too fast within an isthmus

Figure 2.A.1

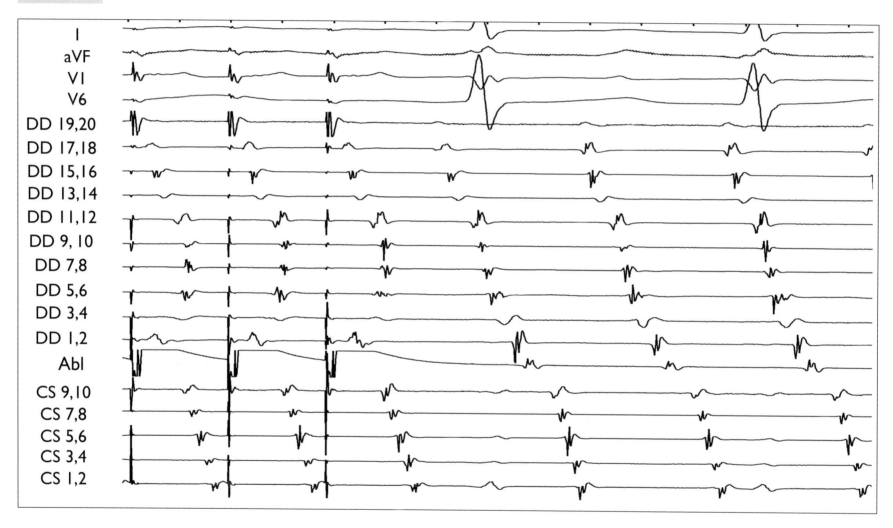

Figure 2.A.2

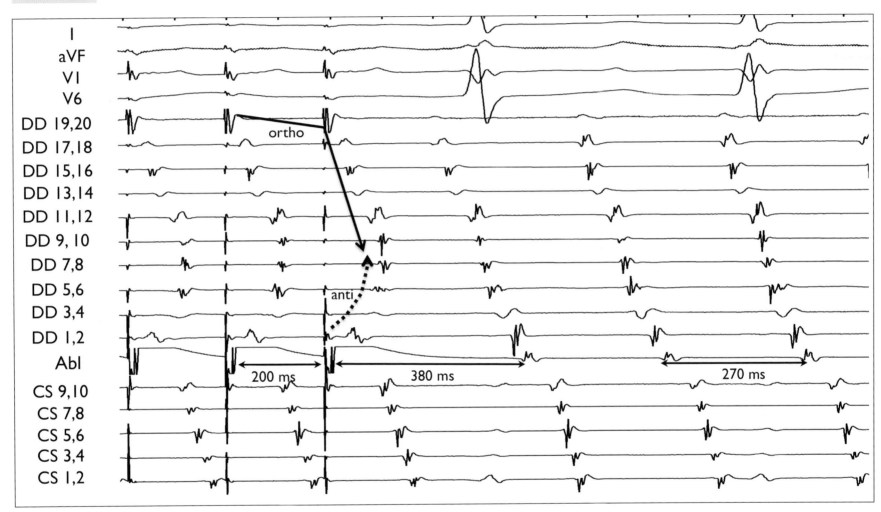

*A*nswer

The correct answer is **D**. This demonstrates entrainment of **typical atrial flutter within the cavotricuspid isthmus**.

The postpacing interval exceeds the tachycardia cycle length (TCL) by over 100 ms, suggesting pacing from a site outside of the circuit. The drive train is 70 ms faster than the TCL, and therefore local conduction delay, or decrement, can prolong the postpacing interval when within a critical isthmus. Deeper penetration of the antidromic wavefront (dashed line) is seen due to faster pacing with collision into DD 7,8, and therefore, intracardiac fusion is present.

The postpacing interval is nearly identical to the TCL when entrainment is performed 20 ms faster than the TCL at the exact same site.

Reference

1. Vollmann D, Stevenson WG, Lüthje L, et al. Misleading long postpacing interval after entrainment of typical atrial flutter from the cavotricuspid isthmus. *J Am Coll Cardiol.* 2012:59(9):819-824.

Figure 2.A.3

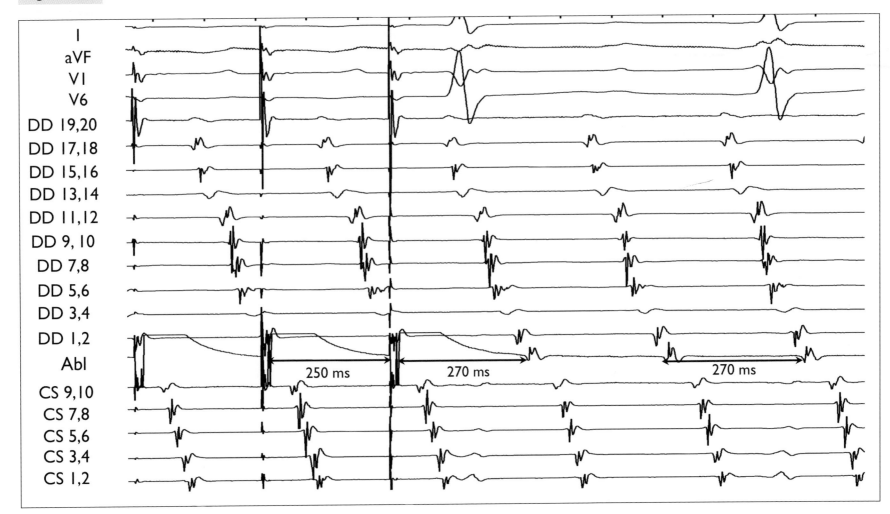

*Q*uestion

What does this pace-mapping response indicate?

A) Failure to capture

B) Fusion

C) Isthmus site

D) Unstable catheter position

Figure 2.B.1

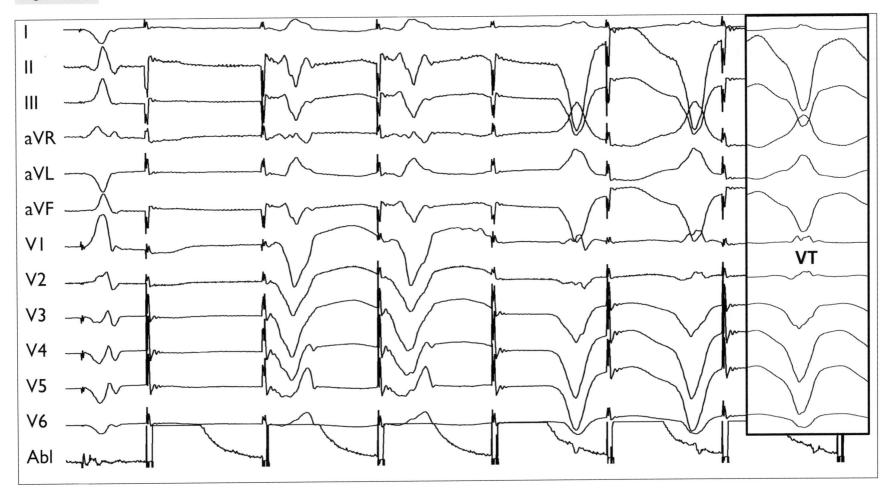

Source: Tung R, Mathuria N, Michowitz Y, et al. Functional pace-mapping responses for identification of targets for catheter ablation of scar-mediated ventricular tachycardia. *Circ Arrhythm Electrophysiol.* 2012;5(2):264-272. With permission.

*A*nswer

The correct answer is **C**. This demonstrates pace-mapping from a site likely to be an **isthmus**.

When multiple morphologies are seen from a single pacing site within scar, this is specific for a central channel with access to multiple exit sites. In this case, pace-mapping from a stable site results in two distinct morphologies with different stimulus latencies. Fusion and failure to capture are not present, as two distinct morphologies follow the first intrinsic pacing complex. The second morphology matches a targeted VT.

Multiple exit sites have been reported in idiopathic VT from focal sources in outflow tracts and papillary muscles. In the setting of scar, the presence of multiple exits has also been shown to account for pleiomorphism and multiple morphologies from the same circuit (common isthmus). This phenomenon illustrates a limitation with pace-mapping where a mismatch can be present at a critical site.

Figure 2.B.2

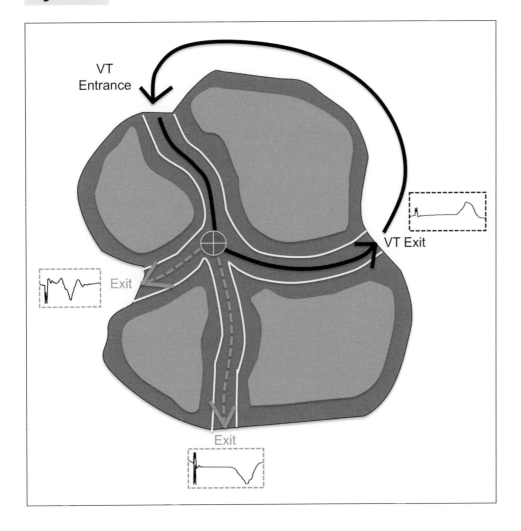

Reference

1. Tung R, Mathuria N, Michowitz Y, et al. Functional pace-mapping responses for identification of targets for catheter ablation of scar-mediated ventricular tachycardia. *Circ Arrhythm Electrophysiol.* 2012;5(2):264-272.

Question

What type of conduction block is shown in this 60-year-old woman with fatigue?

A) Infrahisian block with gap phenomenon

B) AV nodal block with dual physiology

C) AV nodal block

D) Physiologic infrahisian block

Figure 2.C.1

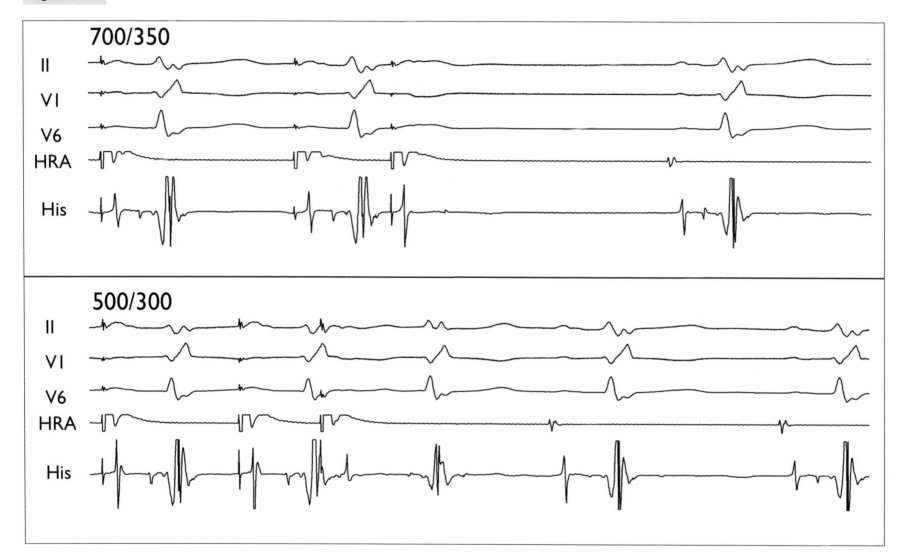

Figure 2.C.2

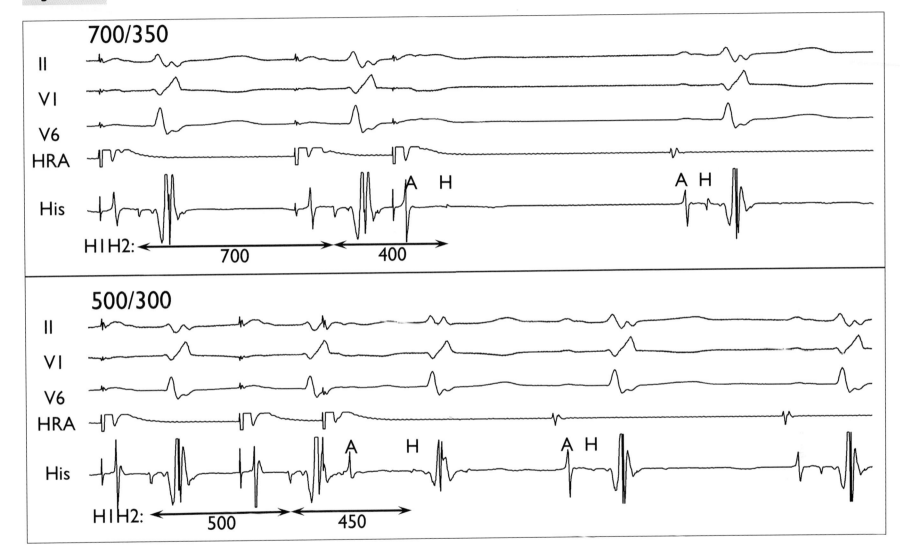

Answer

The correct answer is **A**. Due to slowing in the AV node on the lower tracing, conduction below the His improves as a result of **gap phenomenon**. Gap phenomenon is defined as slowing proximal to a site of conduction block in order to facilitate "paradoxical" distal conduction.

Block in the His-Purkinje system can be physiologic, as it is dependent on the preceding cycle length. In the upper tracing, the block follows a His depolarization, which excludes block in the AV node. The patient has bifascicular block at baseline, which increases the pretest probability of infranodal conduction disease. Normal conduction in the His-Purkinje system is expected to improve at a faster drive cycle and worsen at slower drive cycles (long–short sequences promote infrahisian refractoriness). At first glance, the earlier extrastimulus (350 ms) at a faster drive cycle improves conduction, which favors physiologic infrahisian block.

Importantly, the delay in the AV node (gap) lengthens the effective S2 delivered to the His (450 ms), allowing for conduction below the His. AV nodal block occurred 10 ms faster (500/440 ms). Therefore, there is inadequate "stressing" of the His in this example to discern if block is pathologic or physiologic.

References

1. Kneller J, Shivkumar K, Tung R. Assessment of His–Purkinje reserve: what is the mechanism of block? *Heart Rhythm.* 2012;9(3):465–466.

2. Josephson ME. *Clinical Cardiac Electrophysiology: Techniques and Interpretations,* 4th ed. Philadelphia: Lippincott, Williams & Wilkins, 2008.

Question

What is the mechanism for this run of wide-complex tachycardia?

A) Intermittent preexcitation

B) Ventricular tachycardia

C) Aberration from phase 3 block

D) Aberration from phase 4 block

Figure 2.D.1

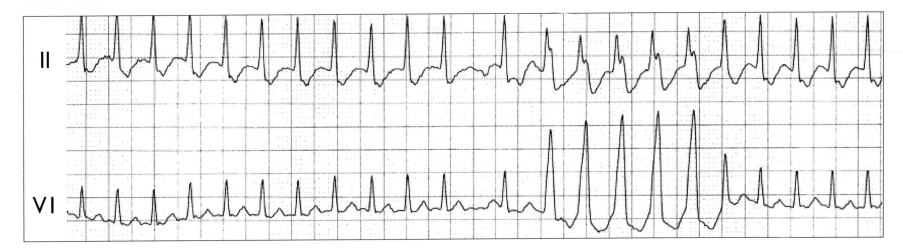

*A*nswer

The correct answer is **C. Phase 3 aberrancy**, or Ashman phenomenon, is seen.

There are four mechanisms of aberrancy: (1) phase 3 block, with physiologic encroachment on the refractory period (tachycardia–related block); (2) phase 4 block from diseased resting membrane potential depolarization during bradycardia; (3) acceleration-dependent block in diseased tissue; and (4) retrograde concealment, where retrograde transseptal penetration perpetuates refractoriness.

The patient is in 1:1 atrial flutter, and the sudden slowing of conduction to 2:1 creates a long–short sequence, which prolongs the expected refractory period of the right bundle branch. The resumption of 1:1 conduction catches the right bundle during phase 3, and aberration occurs. The continuation of aberration occurs due to retrograde concealment of the right bundle via transseptal conduction from the conducted left bundle branch. This is often misinterpreted as nonsustained ventricular tachycardia. Increased preexcitation should not occur after a longer interval, as the AV node can recover excitability, in contrast to the His-Purkinje system. Phase 4 block occurs in the setting of long pauses and bradycardia.

References

1. Gouaux JL, Ashman R. Auricular fibrilation with aberration simulating ventricular paroxysmal tachycardia. *Am Heart J.* 1947;34:366–373.

2. Josephson ME. *Clinical Cardiac Electrophysiology: Techniques and Interpretations,* 4th ed. Philadelphia: Lippincott, Williams & Wilkins, 2008.

Question

What does this pacing maneuver demonstrate in a 40-year-old-man with SVT?

A) Conduction of both AV node and bypass tract

B) Conduction over a bypass tract only

C) Conduction over AV node only

D) Cannot be determined due to atrial capture

Figure 2.E.1

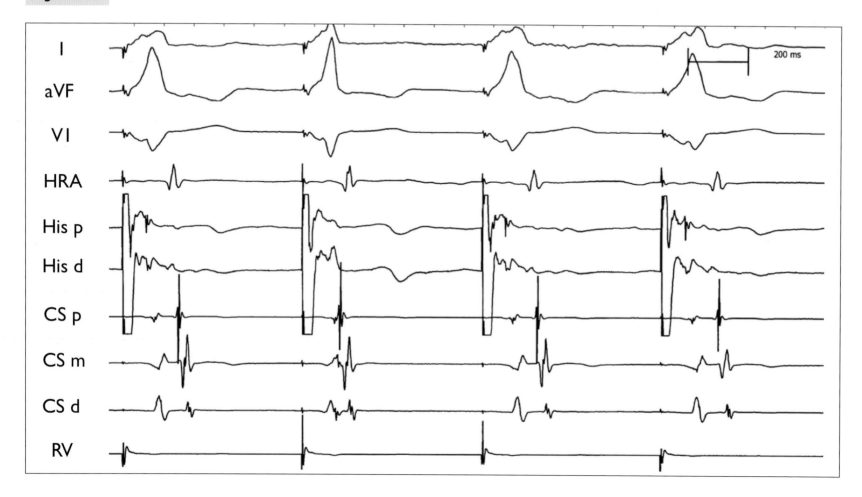

Figure 2.E.2

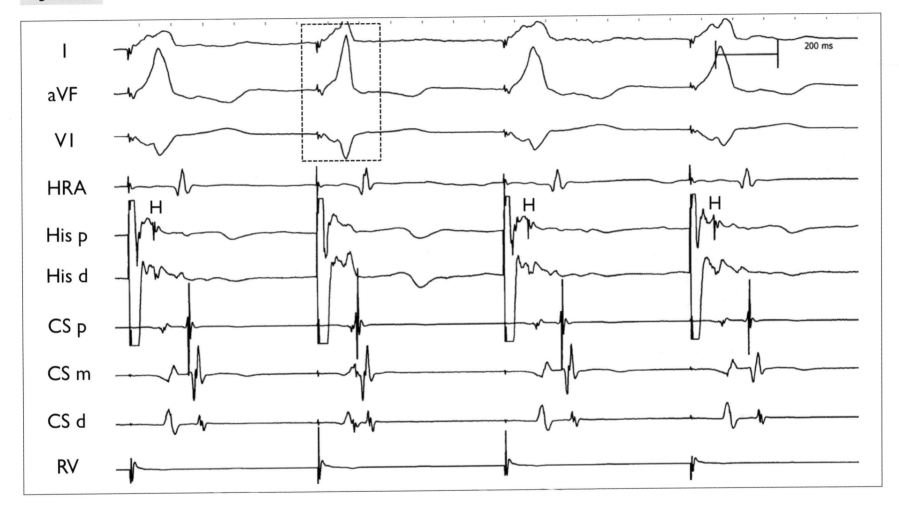

*A*nswer

The correct answer is **C**. Normal retrograde **conduction over the AV node** is shown during parahisian pacing.

Parahisian pacing is performed to detect the presence of retrograde conduction over a bypass tract. Pacing at high output near the His bundle captures both the myocardium and His bundle. Pacing at low output fails to penetrate the insulation of the His bundle and results in capture of the RV myocardium only (wider QRS), which requires more apical engagement of the conduction system, resulting in longer retrograde conduction time in the absence of a bypass tract.

Before interpretation, continuous atrial activation by both narrow (dashed box) and wide complexes should be confirmed. The VA interval is shorter with narrow QRS with His capture (115 ms) compared to the wide QRS without His capture (190 ms). Note the appearance of the His deflection with loss of His capture. This indicates that retrograde activation occurs only over the AV node. Atrial capture is ruled out by the absence of a very short stimulus to atrial timing.

Figure 2.E.3

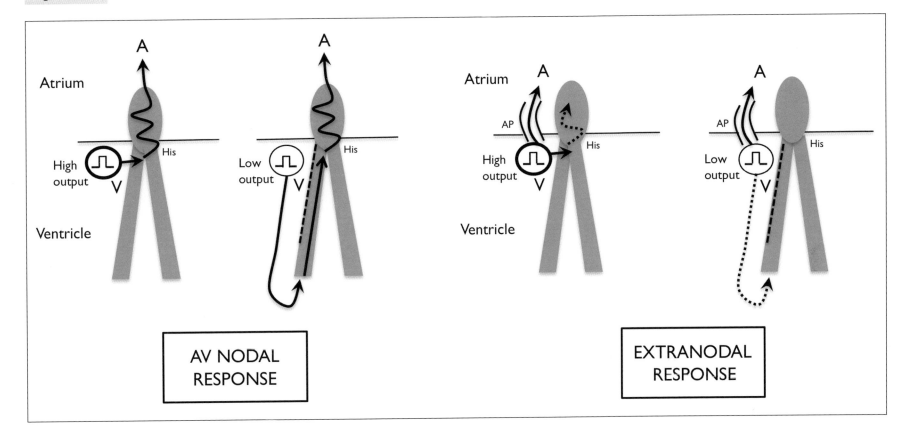

Reference

1. Hirao K, Otomo K, Wang X, et al. Parahisian pacing: A new method for differentiating retrograde conduction over an accessory AV pathway and conduction over the AV node. *Circulation*. 1996;94(5):1027-1035.

Question

What is the most likely mechanism of arrhythmia in a 42-year-old woman?

A) Ventricular tachycardia

B) Mahaim tachycardia

C) Orthodromic reentry using right-sided bypass tract

D) Orthodromic reentry using a left-sided bypass tract

Figure 2.F.1

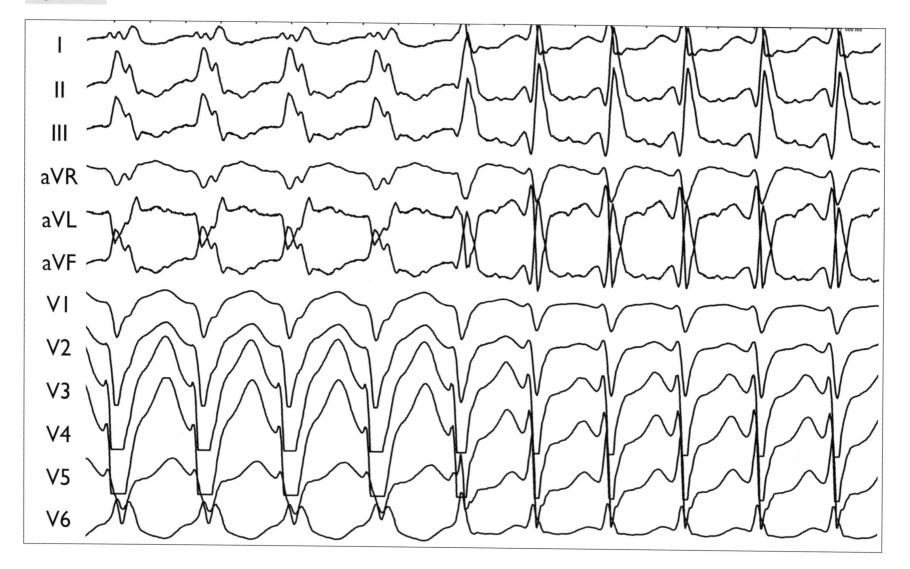

Figure 2.F.2

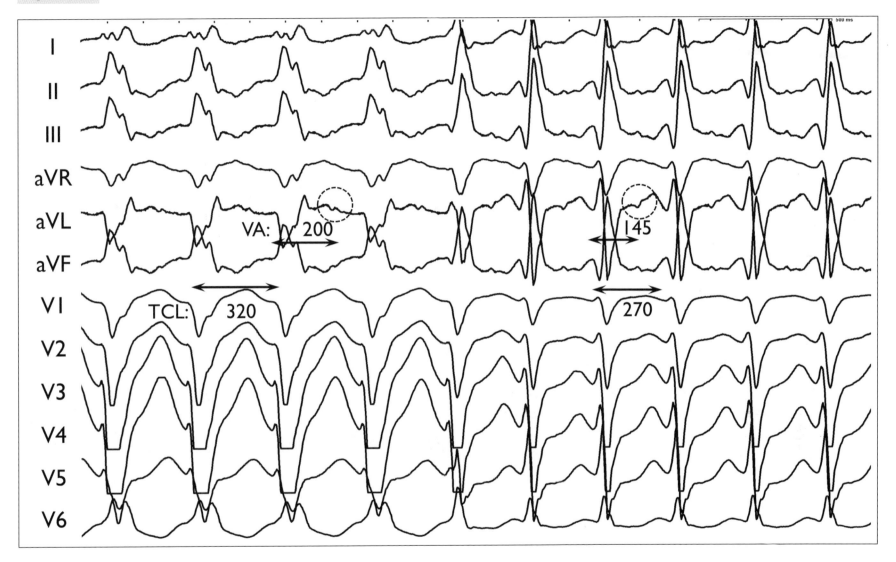

Answer

The correct answer is **D**. Left bundle aberration proves **ortho-dromic reentry using a left-sided bypass tract**.

A wide-complex tachycardia with left bundle branch block morphology (320 ms) is seen transitioning into a more rapid narrow-complex tachycardia (270 ms). VA conduction is consistently seen and the wide-complex tachycardia has a longer VA time (200 ms) than the narrow-complex tachycardia (145 ms). A prolongation of VA time with bundle branch block ipsilateral to a bypass tract is proof of accessory pathway participation in orthodromic tachycardia. The tachycardia cycle does not necessarily prolong in concert with VA prolongation due to changes in AH interval, which can be facilitated with a longer retrograde conduction time.

Mahaim tachycardias (atriofascicular) demonstrate fixed preexcitation and typically exhibit a superior axis. Ventricular tachycardia is a possibility, but does not account for a negative P wave in lead aVL, which is diagnostic of a left-sided atrial pathway insertion.

Reference

1. Josephson ME. *Clinical Cardiac Electrophysiology: Techniques and Interpretations*, 4th ed. Philadelphia: Lippincott, Williams & Wilkins, 2008.

Question

What phenomenon occurs as a result of this pacing maneuver in a 22-year-old man with tachycardia?

A) Change to AVNRT from orthodromic reentry using a concealed right-sided bypass tract

B) Change to AVNRT from orthodromic reentry using a concealed left-sided bypass tract

C) Termination of VT

D) Loss of phase 3 aberration

Figure 2.G.1

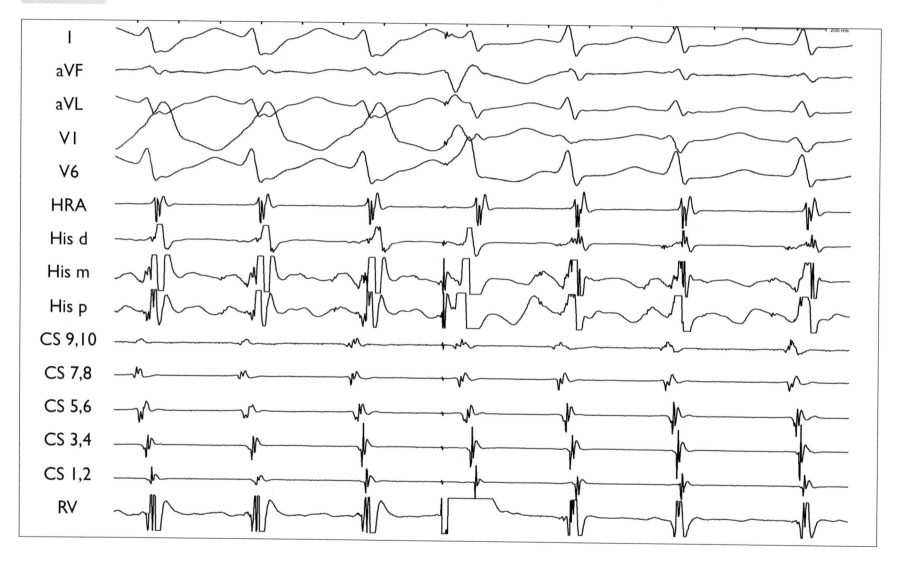

Figure 2.G.2

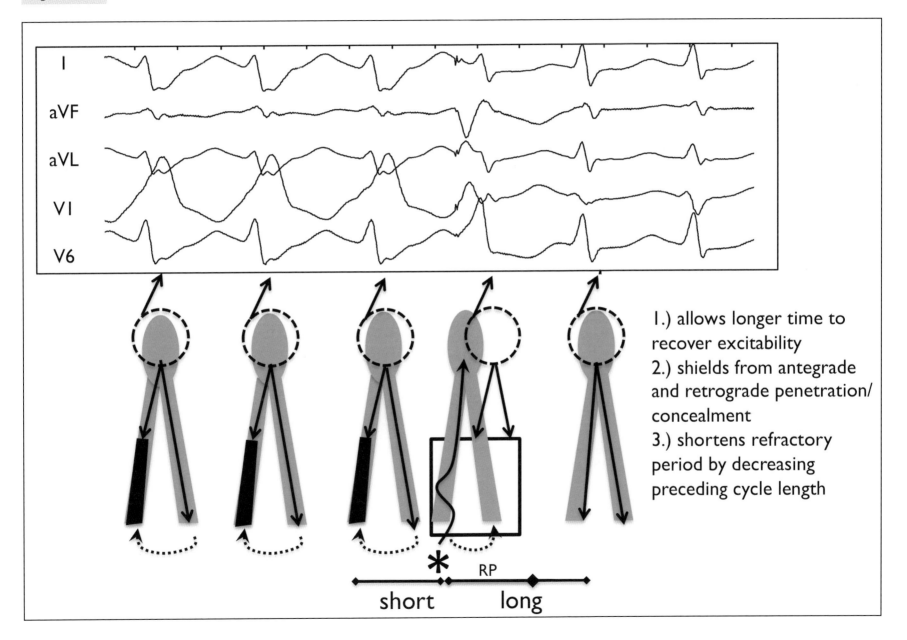

1.) allows longer time to recover excitability

2.) shields from antegrade and retrograde penetration/ concealment

3.) shortens refractory period by decreasing preceding cycle length

*A*nswer

The correct answer is **D. Loss of phase 3 aberration** occurs from this premature ventricular beat.

A wide-complex tachycardia is converted into a narrow-complex tachycardia by a premature ventricular stimulus. The atrial activation sequence is earliest in the His and proximal coronary sinus, and the septal VA timing of <70 ms is specific for AV node reentry. Importantly, the VA interval is unchanged with right bundle, which makes a right-sided pathway unlikely. Ventricular tachycardia is unlikely as the HV interval is the same for both the wide- and narrow-complex tachycardias.

Although the extrastimulus is delivered during His refractoriness, the tracing shows loss of phase 3 aberration by "peeling back" refractoriness. Earlier activation of the right bundle (which is retrogradely concealed) allows for longer time to recover excitability while shielding it from the subsequent tachycardia beat. Importantly, the introduction of a short interval abbreviates the next expectant refractory period, which allows for conduction down the right bundle. While "long–short" intervals promote His-Purkinje refractoriness, this maneuver can be thought of as a "short–long" to facilitate conduction.

Reference

1. Josephson ME. *Clinical Cardiac Electrophysiology: Techniques and Interpretations,* 4th ed. Philadelphia: Lippincott, Williams & Wilkins, 2008.

Question

During atrial pacing, the following is observed in a 60-year-old woman with presyncope. What is the next step based on this tracing?

A) Repeat pacing with atropine

B) Repeat pacing with isoproterenol

C) Implant dual-chamber pacemaker

D) No additional testing or intervention

Figure 2.H.1

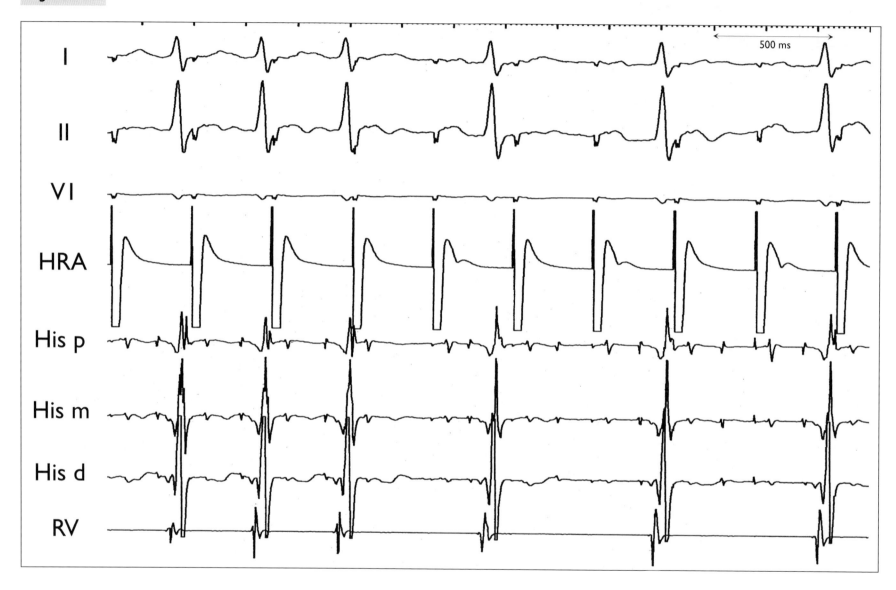

Figure 2.H.2

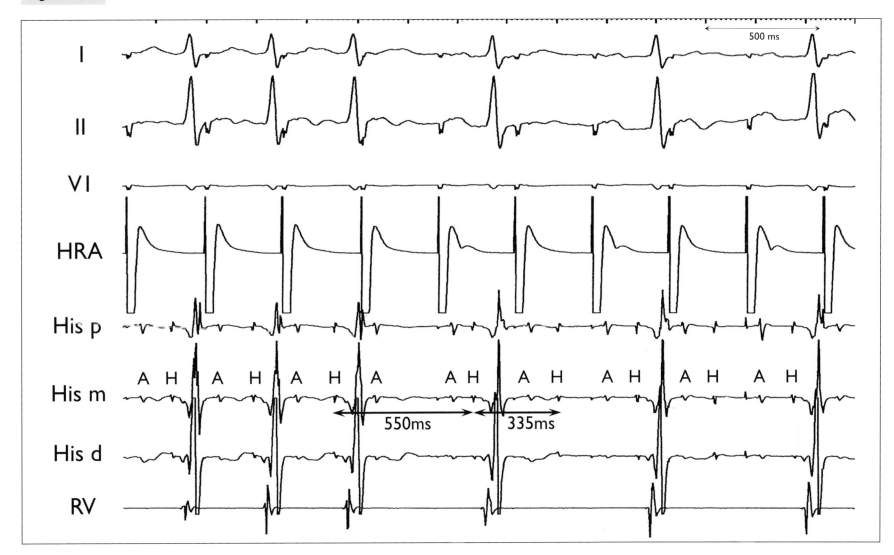

Answer

The correct answer is **D. Physiologic infrahisian block** is seen during rapid atrial pacing.

In this tracing, the atrium is paced at a cycle length of 300 ms. The first three atrial paced beats are conducted to the ventricle with progressive prolongation of AH interval, followed by block in the AV node (Wenckebach, Mobitz type I). The next atrial paced beat (fifth beat) is conducted due to recovery in the AV node. This sets up an input to the His as a "long–short" interval (550/335 ms). Because the refractoriness of the His-Purkinje system is dependent on the preceding diastolic interval or cycle length, the increase in refractoriness results in Mobitz type II infrahisian block (sixth beat). This leads to a repeated long–short cycle lengths, resulting in a "locked in" 2:1 phase III infrahisian block of both bundles.

Atropine and isoproterenol improve conduction through the AV node, but do not improve infrahisian block. Increasing refractoriness due to a prolonged preceding diastolic interval is normal physiologic behavior of the His-Purkinje system and does not indicate the need for a dual-chamber pacemaker.

References

1. Denes P, Wu D, Dhingra R, Pietras RJ, Rosen KM. The effects of cycle length on cardiac refractory periods in man. *Circulation.* 1974;49:32–41.

2. Denker S, Shenasa M, Gilbert CJ, Akhtar M. Effects of abrupt changes in cycle length on refractoriness of the His-Purkinje system in man. *Circulation.* 1983;67:60–68.

3. Josephson ME. *Clinical Cardiac Electrophysiology: Techniques and Interpretations,* 4th ed. Philadelphia: Lippincott, Williams & Wilkins, 2008.

Question

What is demonstrated by this pacing maneuver in a 21-year-old man with recurrent palpitations?

A) Retrograde conduction over AV node

B) Retrograde conduction over bypass tract

C) Retrograde conduction over two bypass tracts

D) Cannot be determined

Figure 2.I.1

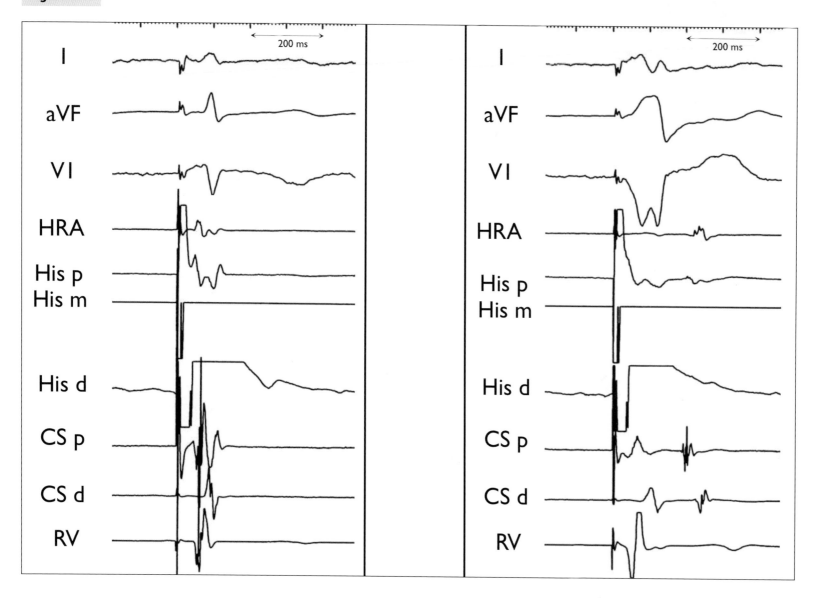

Figure 2.1.2

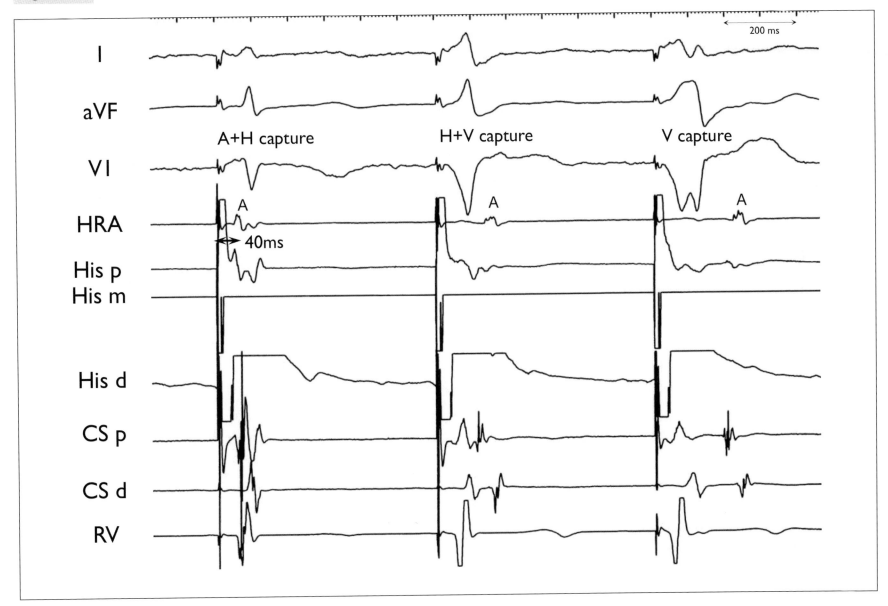

Answer

The correct answer is **D. Interpretation of parahisian pacing is limited** by atrial capture.

In this case, the first beat is narrow (His capture), and the second beat is wide (loss of His capture). When a pathway is proven by parahisian pacing, the VA times are the same, as retrograde conduction is independent of His activation. An interpretation of a nodal response to this maneuver is suggested by a shorter VA time with narrow complex, and VA prolongation with the wider complex. However, the atrial activation occurs within 40 ms of the stimulus. Such a short conduction time (stimulus to HRA <70 ms, or stimulus to coronary sinus <60 ms) is unlikely if the atrial activation occurs over the AV node, or even a septal pathway. The atrium is activated directly due to high-output pacing, rendering this maneuver uninterpretable. The maneuver should be repeated after catheter repositioning or decreasing the pacing output.

Analysis of an interposed beat adequately demonstrates a nodal response. The first beat shows direct atrial and His capture. The second beat results in capture of the His and ventricle (wider), and the third beat is only ventricular capture (widest). The activation sequence in the second and third beats is the same over the AV node; only the stimulus to atrium interval changes.

References

1. Hirao K, Otomo K, Wang X, et al. Parahisian pacing: A new method for differentiating retrograde conduction over an accessory AV pathway and conduction over the AV node. *Circulation*. 1996;94(5):1027-1035.
2. Obeyesekere M, Leong-Sit P, Skanes A, et al. Determination of inadvertent atrial capture during para-Hisian pacing. *Circ Arrhythm Electrophysiol*. 2011;4:510-514.

Case 2.J

Question

How is the mechanism of the variable heart rate during atrial flutter best explained?

A) AV nodal Wenckebach

B) Infranodal block

C) Intrahisian block

D) Multilevel block in AV node

Figure 2.J.1

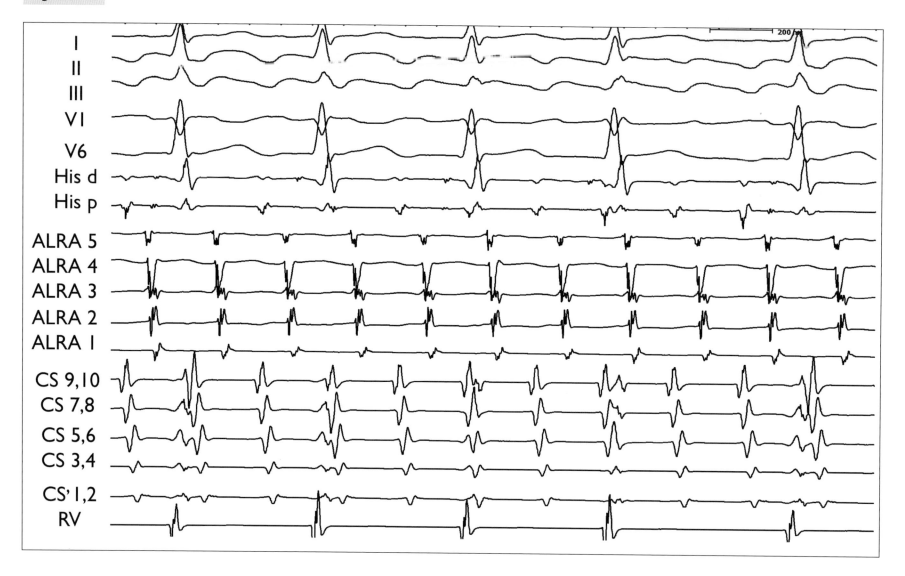

Figure 2.J.2

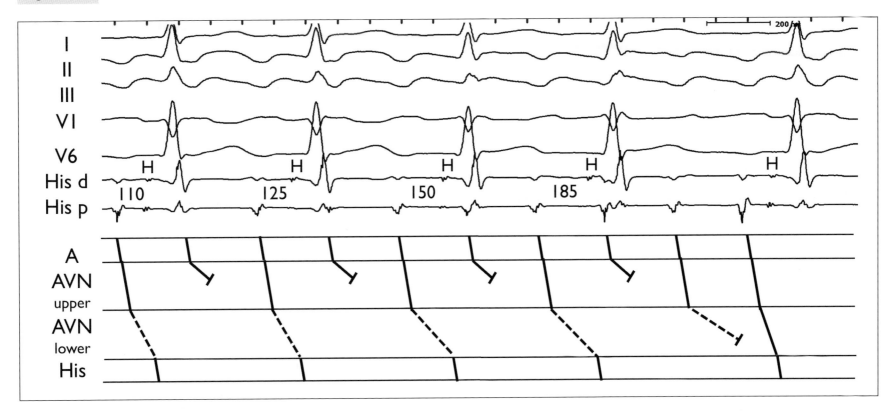

*A*nswer

The correct answer is **D**. The progression of 3:1 block from 2:1 block during typical atrial flutter is best explained by **multilevel block in the AV node**.

The level of block within in the AV node as a His deflection is absent during each nonconducted beat. The presence of a His electrogram would signify intrahisian or infrahisian block (Mobitz II). Wenckebach in the AV node is seen on every other beat (alternating Wenckebach), which implies that two levels of block are present. Multilevel block within the AV node with fixed 2:1 block at one level and Wenckebach at another level best accounts for the progression to 3:1 block. The presence of a repetitive variable conduction sequence suggests multilevel block that is physiologic.

References

1. Slama R, Leclerq JF, Rosengarten M, Coumel P, Bourvrain Y. Multilevel block in the atrioventricular node during atrial tachycardia and flutter alternating with Wenckebach phenomenon. *Br Heart J.* 1979;42(4):463-470.

2. Castellanos A, Interian A, Cox MM, Myerburg RJ. Alternating Wenckebach periods and allied arrhythmias. *Pacing Clin Electrophysiol.* 1993;16(12):2285-2300.

Question

What does this response to a pacing maneuver in a 30-year-old woman with supraventricular tachycardia demonstrate?

A) Non-capture/pseudo-fusion

B) AV nodal response

C) Presence of accessory pathway

D) Atrial capture

Figure 2.K.1

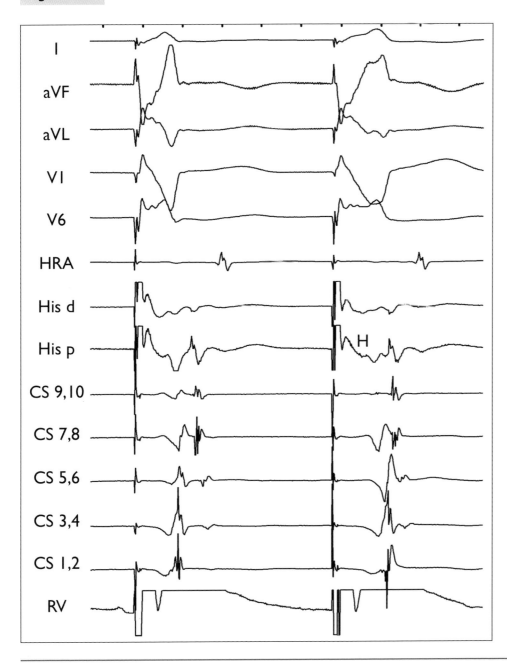

*A*nswer

The correct answer is **C**. An extranodal response to parahisian pacing demonstrates the **presence of an accessory pathway**.

Pacing from the basal right ventricle is seen on surface QRS morphology. At a high pacing output, the first complex is narrower than the second, indicating capture of the His bundle. The emergence of a retrograde His potential is seen upon loss of capture on the second paced complex, where the local ventricular activation in the coronary sinus is delayed, with a fixed stimulus to atrium timing.

The VA time and retrograde activation sequence is unchanged despite loss of His capture, indicating that an extranodal connection between the atrium and ventricle is present. In the absence of a pathway, loss of His bundle capture requires myocardial conduction down to the apex to access the His-Purkinje system in a retrograde fashion, which results in a longer VA conduction time. Atrial capture is ruled out by the absence of a very short stimulus-to-atrial timing.

Reference

1.   Hirao K, Otomo K, Wang X, et al. Parahisian pacing. A new method for differentiating retrograde conduction over an accessory AV pathway from conduction over the AV node. *Circulation*. 1996;94(5):1027-1035.

*Q*uestion

A pacing maneuver is performed in a 32-year-old man with recurrent palpitations. Why are the results different?

A) Site of pacing

B) Multiple pathways

C) Timing of extrastimulus

D) Two tachycardia mechanisms

Figure 2.L.1

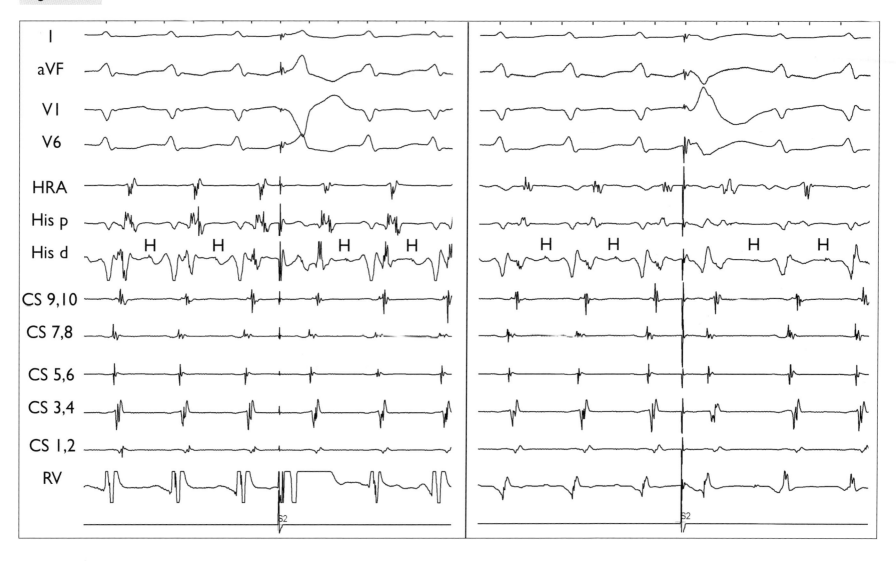

*A*nswer

The correct answer is **A**. The ability to advance the atrial activation during tachycardia is dependent upon the **site of pacing**.

The earliest atrial activation during supraventricular tachycardia is CS 7,8, suggestive of an orthodromic tachycardia utilizing a left posteroseptal pathway. There is no change in tachycardia before and after the pacing maneuver, and both PVCs are synchronous with His activation. The His-refractory PVC from the right ventricle (left bundle branch block morphology) does not affect the atrium during tachycardia. This would suggest the absence of an accessory pathway. However, a PVC delivered from the left ventricle (right bundle branch morphology) is closer to the ventricular insertion site of the pathway and advances the atrial activation.

This case highlights the fact that His-refractory PVCs can never be used to exclude the presence of a pathway. This maneuver is only useful to prove the presence of an accessory pathway when the atrial activation is advanced. The advanced atrial activation sequence is identical to the activation during tachycardia, which is strongly suggestive of participation rather than a bystander. There is no evidence of multiple pathway activation sequences.

Reference

1. Josephson ME. *Clinical Cardiac Electrophysiology: Techniques and Interpretations,* 4th ed. Philadelphia: Lippincott, Williams & Wilkins, 2008.

Case 2.M

Question

Which of the following is shown during ablation of the mitral isthmus?

A) Unidirectional block

B) Bidirectional block

C) Conduction slowing without block

D) None of the above

Figure 2.M.1

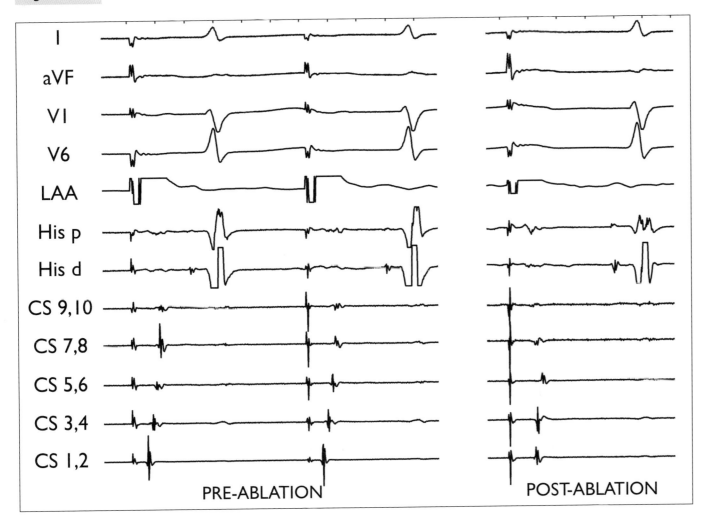

PRE-ABLATION

POST-ABLATION

Figure 2.M.2

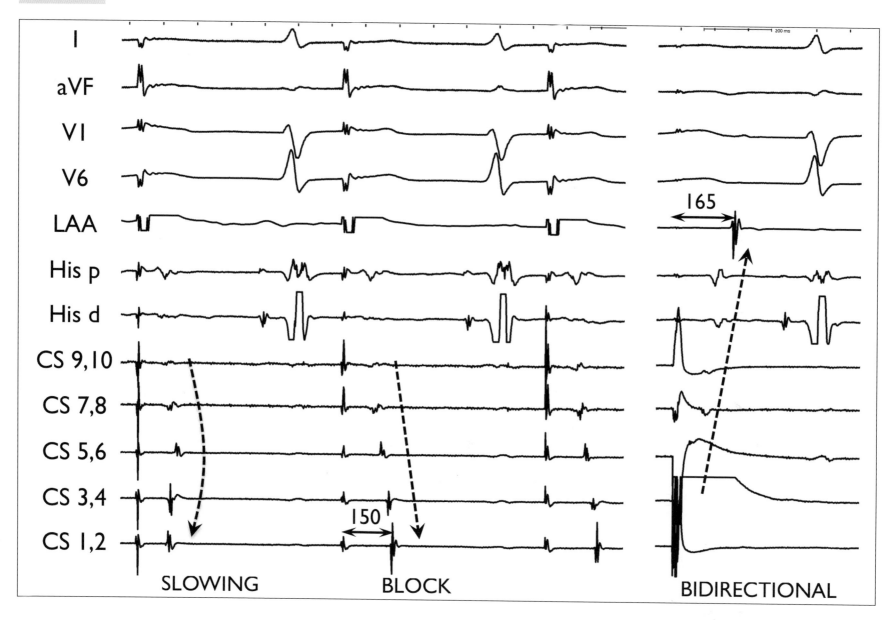

Figure 2.M.3

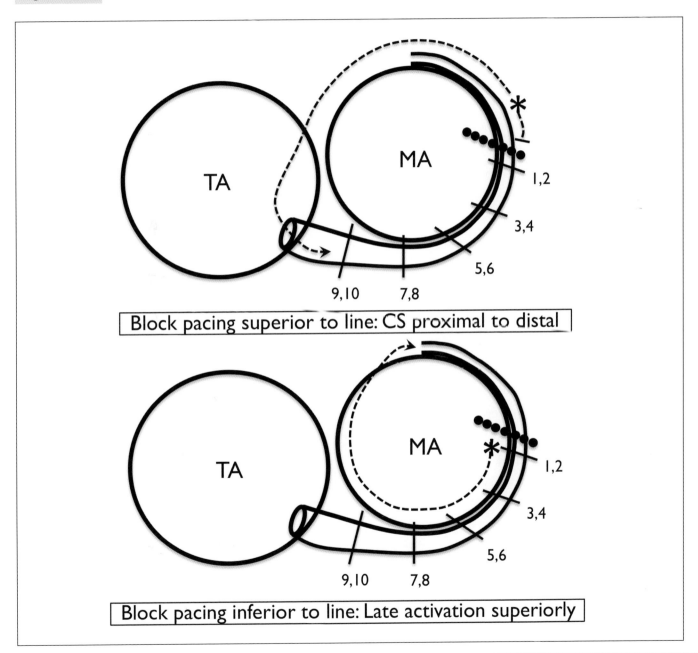

Block pacing superior to line: CS proximal to distal

Block pacing inferior to line: Late activation superiorly

*A*nswer

The correct answer is **C. Conduction slowing without block** across the mitral isthmus is shown.

The targeted endpoint of linear ablation across the mitral isthmus is bidirectional block. Unidirectional block is demonstrated when pacing anterior and superior (left atrial appendage) to the ablation line shows proximal to distal activation in the coronary sinus (CS). Pacing inferior to the line with a similarly long conduction time is required to demonstrate bidirectional block. Differential pacing from CS electrodes can be also performed to demonstrate a shorter activation time when pacing farther away from the line of block.

Several pitfalls can be present when testing for mitral isthmus block, where block can be misinterpreted to be present or absent. In this example, pacing from the left atrial appendage shows a change in CS activation, although activation to CS 1,2 is still simultaneous with CS 9,10, demonstrating slow conduction across the ablation line. When complete block is achieved, activation shows latest activation in CS 1,2 (150 ms). Bidirectional block is shown pacing from CS 3,4 (165 ms). Careful distinction between epicardial CS potentials and far-field endocardial left atrial electrograms also must be made when assessing for mitral isthmus block.

References

1. Jaïs P, Hocini M, Hsu LF, et al. Technique and results of linear ablation at the mitral isthmus. *Circulation*. 2004;110(19):2996-3002.

2. Shah AJ, Pascale P, Miyazaki S, et al. Prevalence and types of pitfall in the assessment of mitral isthmus linear conduction block. *Circ Arrhythm Electrophysiol*. 2012;5(5):957-967.

PART 3

Intracardiac Tracings

Question

What does this entrainment response demonstrate?

A) Inner loop

B) Outer loop

C) Isthmus

D) Dead-end bystander

Figure 3.A.1

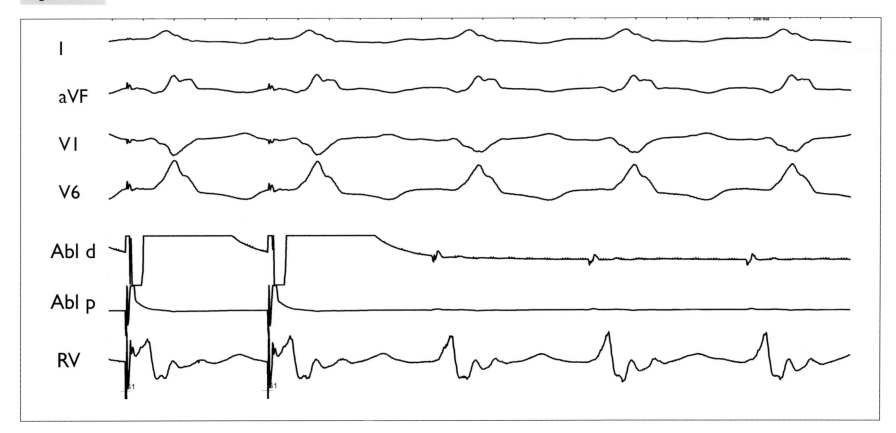

Figure 3.A.2

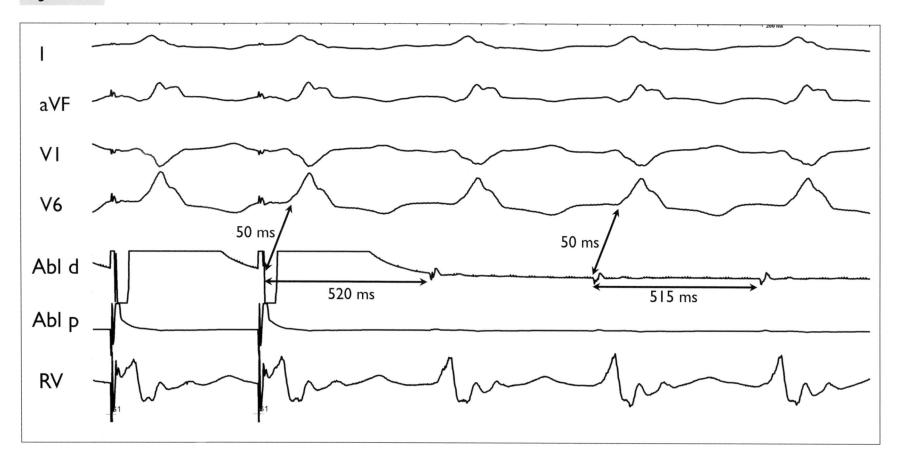

Figure 3.A.3

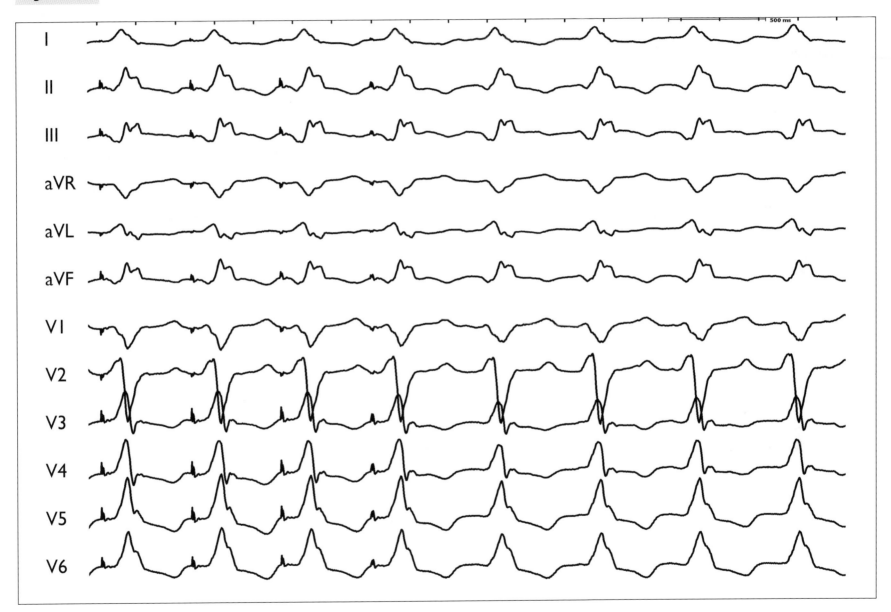

Answer

The correct answer is **C**. Demonstration of an **isthmus** is shown.

Three criteria must be fulfilled at an isthmus site: (1) post-pacing interval (PPI) within 30 ms of the tachycardia cycle length; (2) concealed fusion (antidromic collision within a protected site with orthodromic exit identical to VT); and (3) stimulus to QRS (S-QRS) equal to EGM-QRS interval.

Concealed fusion is seen during entrainment with a 12/12 match with the VT. Outer loop sites and remote bystanders exhibit manifest fusion. Dead-end bystander and inner loop sites have long S-QRS and EGM-QRS intervals. Dead-end bystander sites that are attached to the circuit show concealed fusion but have a long PPI response. As the PPI is nearly identical to the TCL, and the S-QRS and EGM-QRS intervals are the same in this case, an isthmus site (distal close to exit, EGM-QRS <30% of TCL) is demonstrated. Ablation at this site resulted in abrupt termination of ventricular tachycardia.

References

1. Stevenson WG, Khan H, Sager P, et al. Identification of reentry circuit sites during catheter mapping and radiofrequency ablation of ventricular tachycardia late after myocardial infarction. *Circulation.* 1993;88:1647-1670.

2. El-Shalakany A, Hadjis T, Papageorgiou P, Monahan K, Epstein L, Josephson ME. Entrainment/mapping criteria for the prediction of termination of ventricular tachycardia by single radiofrequency lesion in patients with coronary artery disease. *Circulation.* 1999;99(17):2283-2289.

Question

What does this entrainment response demonstrate?

A) Remote bystander

B) Outer loop

C) Isthmus

D) Dead-end bystander

Figure 3.B.1

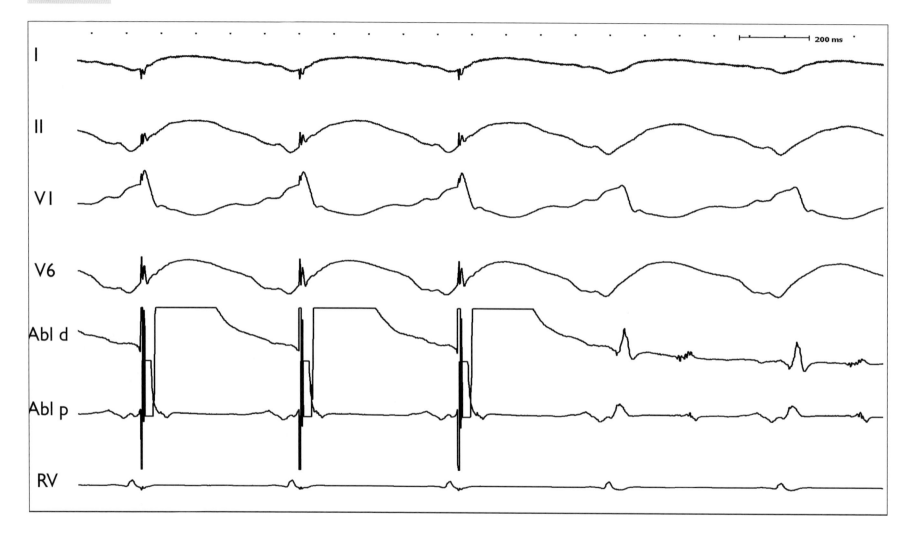

Figure 3.B.2

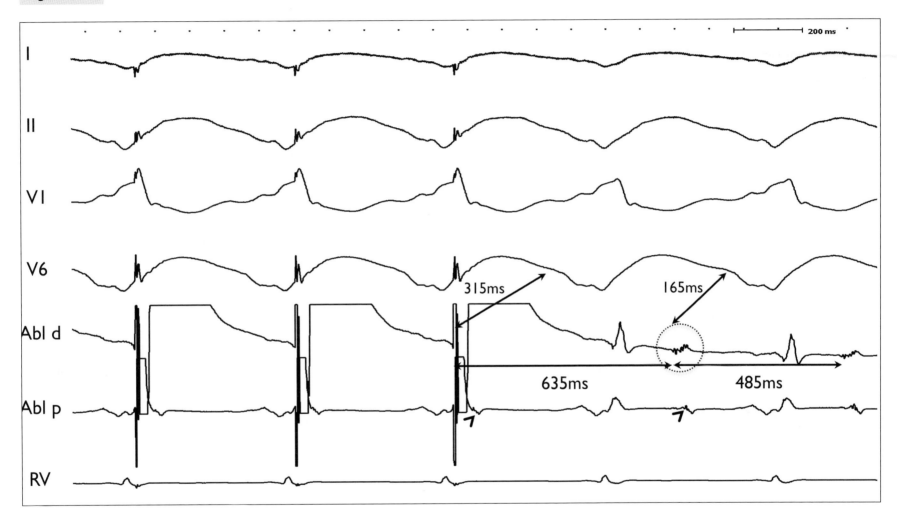

Answer

The correct answer is **D**. This demonstrates **entrainment of a "dead-end" bystander**.

When assessing the entrainment response to identify location in the circuit, three questions must be asked and answered:

1. Is there manifest (overt) or concealed fusion?

2. What is the PPI-TCL difference?

3. Are the S-QRS and EGM-QRS the same?

Myocardial capture must first be confirmed when concealed fusion is suspected (a common pitfall), and then an analysis of which component of the local electrogram was captured should be undertaken.

In this patient, there are two local electrograms sensed on the distal electrode, and the more fractionated, low-amplitude signal appears "near-field." Capture of this local electrogram (circle) is evidenced by the disappearance of it during pacing. Note that the terminal portion of this electrogram (arrowhead) is seen on the proximal ablation electrode immediately after the pacing stimulus artifact.

Concealed fusion is present, indicating that the site of pacing is within or attached to the reentrant circuit, which rules out a remote bystander and an outer loop site. Beware of the pacing stimulus artifact that distorts the surface QRS morphology in V_1.

The S-QRS exceeds the EGM-QRS ($315 - 165 = 150$ ms) by the same difference between the PPI and TCL ($635 - 485 = 150$ ms) in a dead-end bystander, as there is additional time required to "pace out of" and "sense into" the bystander.

Figure 3.B.3

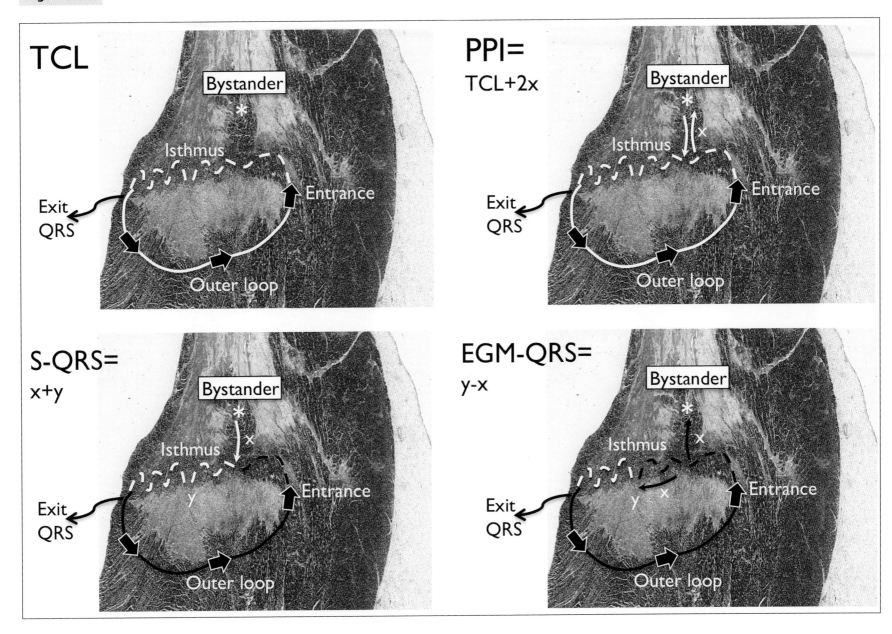

Reference

1. Stevenson WG, Khan H, Sager P, et al. Identification of reentry circuit sites during catheter mapping and radiofrequency ablation of ventricular tachycardia late after myocardial infarction. *Circulation*. 1993;88:1647-1670.

2. Almendral JM, Gottlieb CD, Rosenthal ME, et al. Entrainment of ventricular tachycardia: explanation for surface electrocardiographic phenomena by analysis of electrograms recorded within the tachycardia circuit. *Circulation*. 1988;77:569-580.

Question

Where is the site of block in this 65-year-old woman presenting with lightheadedness?

A) AV node

B) Intra-His

C) Infra-His

D) Sinoatrial

Figure 3.C.1

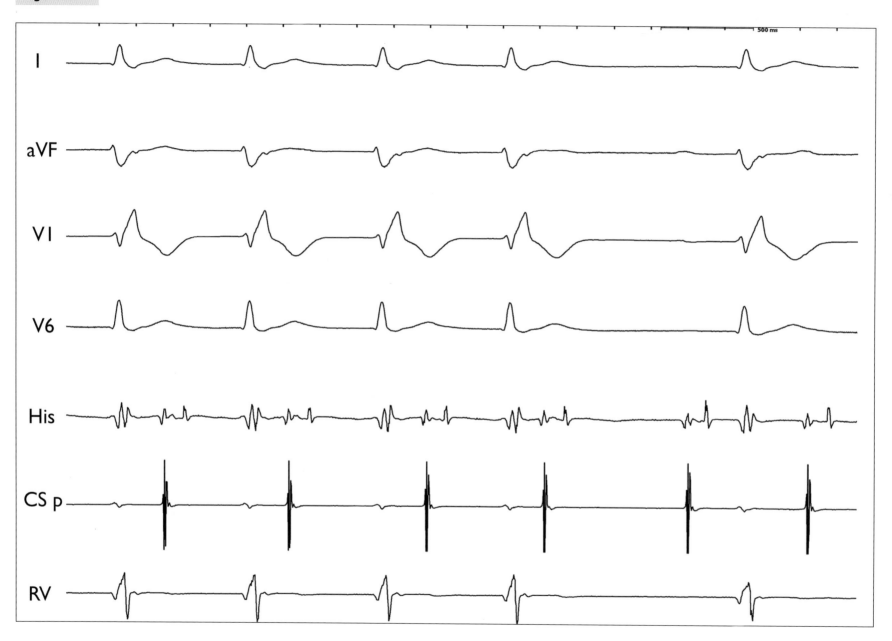

Figure 3.C.2

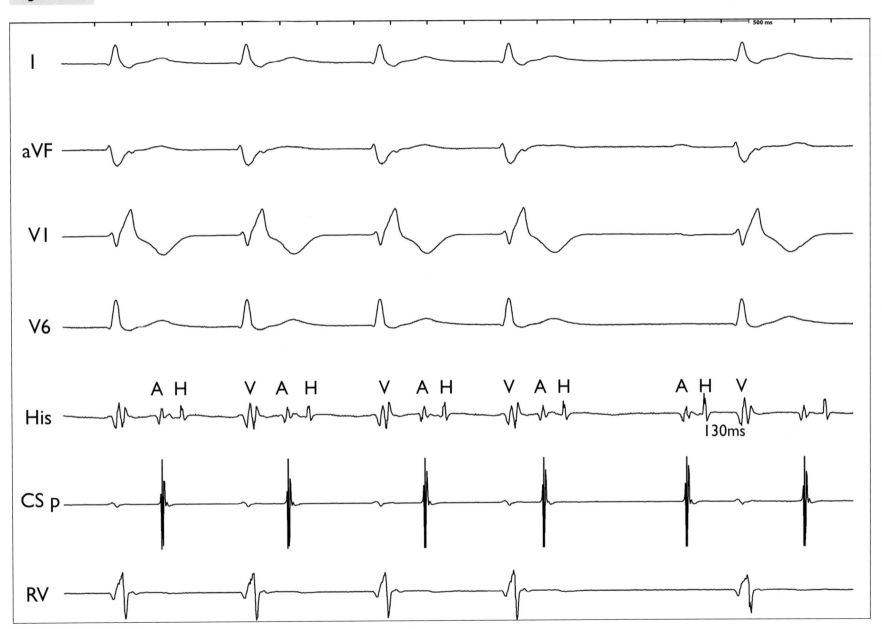

*A*nswer

The correct answer is **C**. The level of block is **infrahisian**.

The baseline 12-lead ECG shows His–Purkinje disease with right bundle branch block and left anterior fascicular block, raising the pretest probability of infranodal block.

Wenckebach is most commonly seen in the AV node, but in rare cases, a diseased His–Purkinje system can exhibit decremental conduction prior to block. When the PR interval is extremely long, the AH is typically much more prolonged than the HV. In this patient, the AH interval remains constant with significant HV conduction delay until block is seen after the His depolarization. The return beat after block shows a shorter, baseline HV interval (130 ms). With extreme PR prolongation, the P wave may be difficult to identify, as it falls in the T wave.

Reference

1.   Josephson ME. *Clinical Cardiac Electrophysiology: Techniques and Interpretations*, 4th ed. Philadelphia: Lippincott, Williams & Wilkins, 2008.

Question

What does this entrainment response demonstrate?

A) Remote bystander

B) Outer loop

C) Isthmus

D) Cannot be determined

Figure 3.D.1

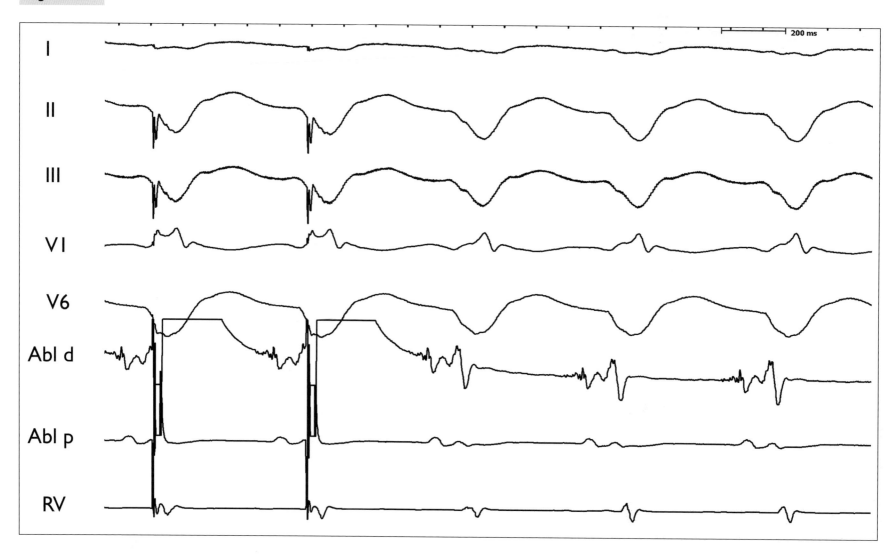

Figure 3.D.2

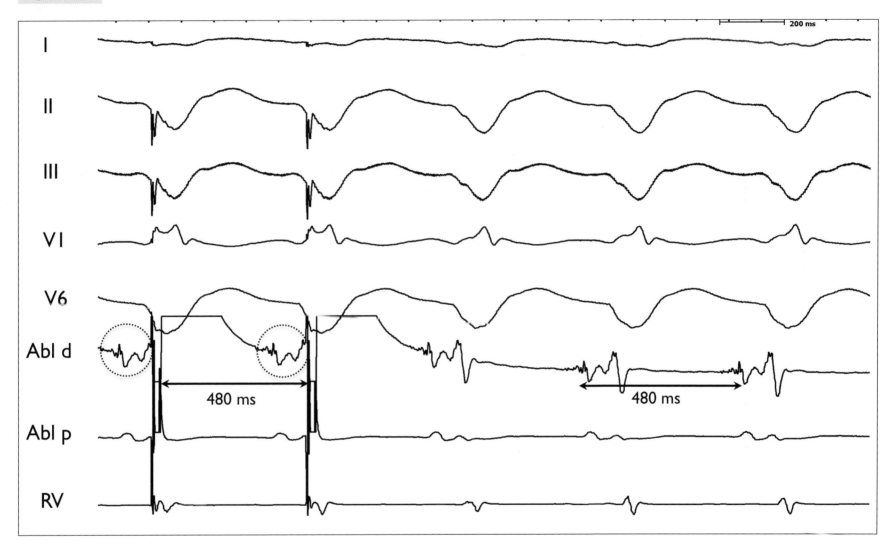

Answer

The correct answer is **D**. This demonstrates **failure to capture due to pacing too close to the tachycardia cycle length (TCL)**.

Two clues are present to indicate failure to capture: (1) The stimulus is within the QRS, which would necessitate capture of the following QRS. This S–QRS would be extremely long and close to the TCL (480 ms). (2) The onset of both local electrograms (circled) is seen during pacing at 480 ms, indicating that they are not captured or far-field.

If attempts at entrainment appear to show concealed fusion on surface morphology, as in this case, capture of a local electrogram must be confirmed. When pacing close to the TCL, pacing for entrainment often needs to be repeated at a slightly faster rate or for a longer duration to ensure adequate and consistent capture.

Reference

1. Issa ZF, Miller JM, Zipes DP. *Clinical Arrhythmology and Electrophysiology*, 2nd ed. Philadelphia: Elsevier, 2012:chap 22.

Question

What type of pathway is shown in this 32-year-old woman with palpitations?

A) Anteroseptal bypass tract

B) Mahaim atriofascicular

C) Fasciculoventricular

D) Right free wall bypass tract

Figure 3.E.1

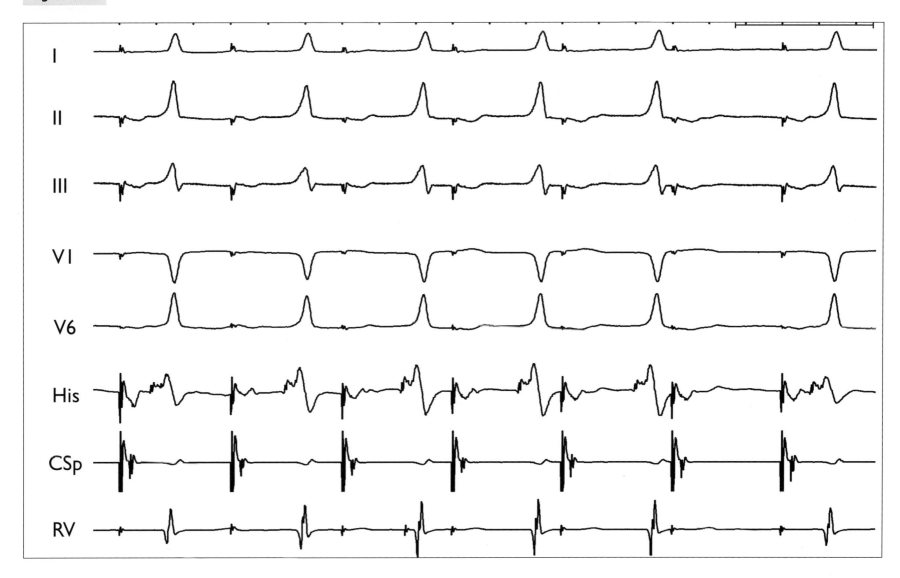

Figure 3.E.2

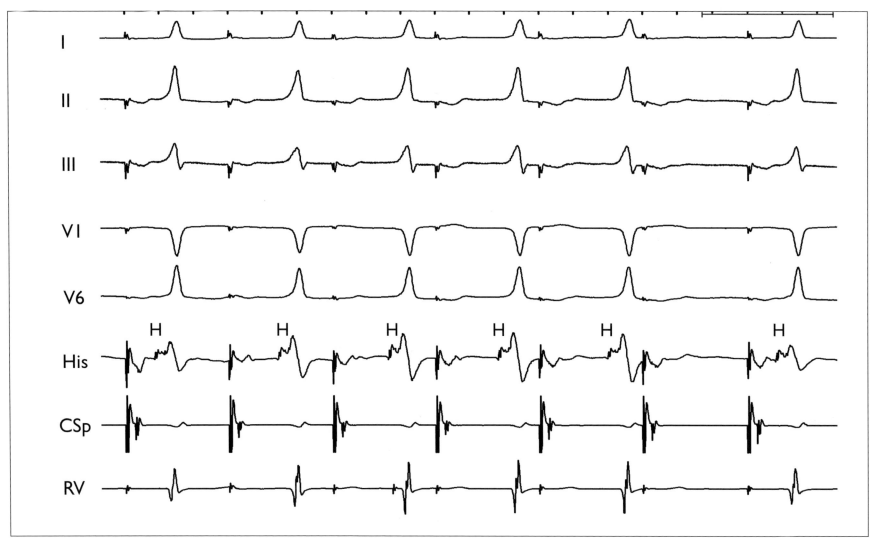

Source for Figures 3.E.1 and 3.E.2: Tung R, Sklyar E, Josephson M. An unusual form of preexcitation: fasciculoventricular bypass tract. *Heart Rhythm*. 2008;5(12):1767-1768. With permission from Elsevier.

Figure 3.E.3

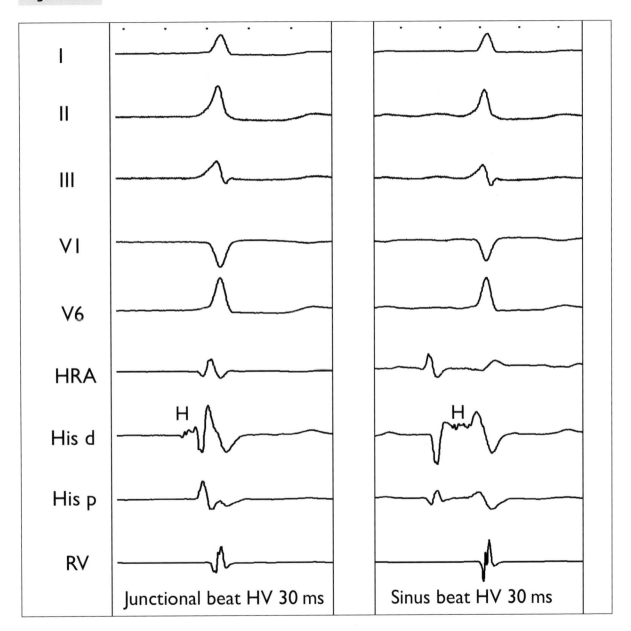

Answer

The correct answer is **C**. This demonstrates the presence of a **fasciculoventricular bypass tract**.

Several unique features of this type of bypass tract are seen. There is minimal preexcitation at baseline. Fixed rather than progressive preexcitation is seen during burst atrial pacing with AV nodal decrement, as conduction must occur through the AV node to reach the distal bypass tract. Mahaim bypass tracts exhibit increasing preexcitation with variable degrees of decrement in the pathway with burst pacing. Importantly, a junctional beat will manifest the same fixed preexcitation (HV 30 ms) in contrast to atrioventricular bypass tracts.

The delta-wave pattern appears similar to anteroseptal bypass tracts, as the insertion is below His. Fasciculoventricular bypass tracts do not result in clinical tachycardia, and ablation is not indicated.

References

1. Tung R, Sklyar E, Josephson ME. An unusual form of preexcitation: fasciculoventricular bypass tract. *Heart Rhythm*. 2008;5(12):1767-1768.

2. Josephson ME. *Clinical Cardiac Electrophysiology: Techniques and Interpretations*, 4th ed. Philadelphia: Lippincott, Williams & Wilkins, 2008.

Question

What is the mechanism of tachycardia?

A) Sinus rhythm with dual AV node response

B) Ventricular tachycardia

C) Junctional bigeminy

D) AVNRT with block to atrium

Figure 3.F.1

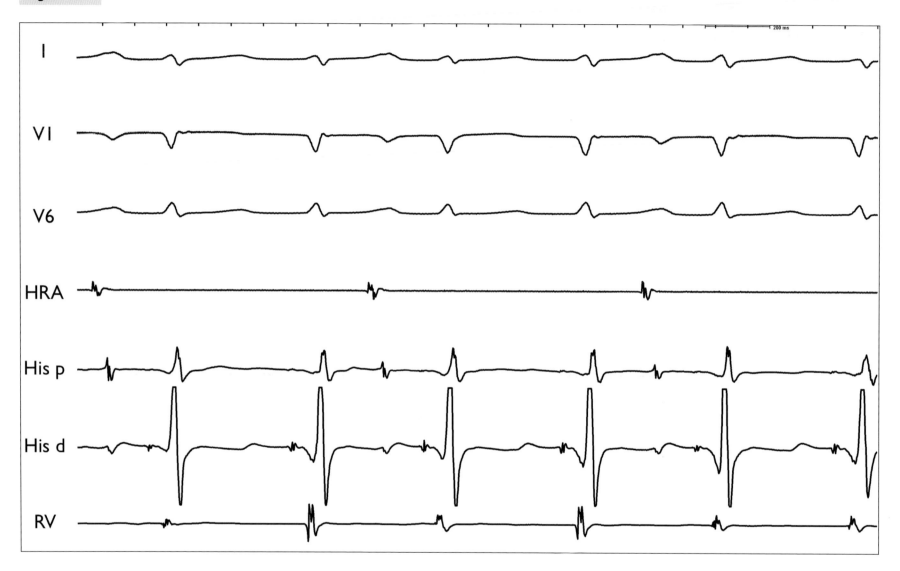

Figure 3.F.2

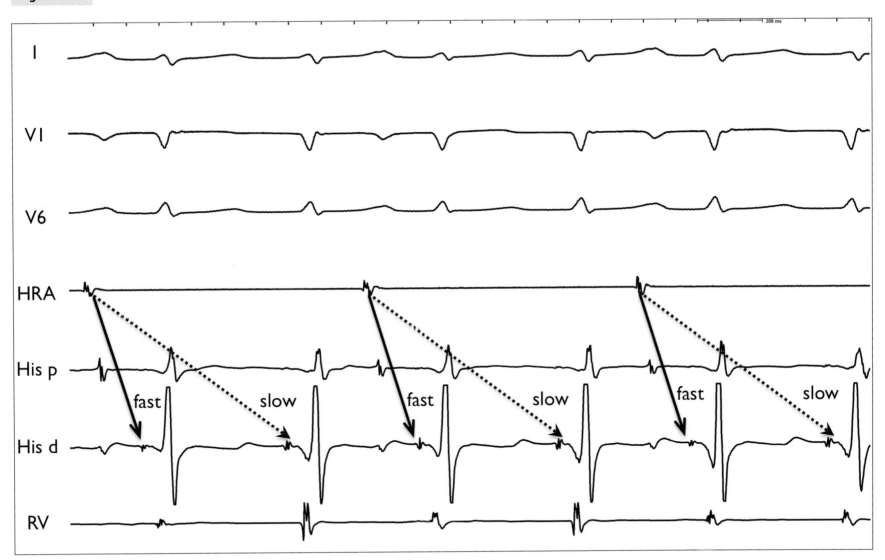

Answer

The correct answer is **A. A "2-for-1" response or "double fire" in normal sinus rhythm** is shown.

When there are more ventricular events than atrial events, ventricular tachycardia and junctional tachycardia with VA dissociation should be considered. A His precedes each narrow QRS, which makes ventricular tachycardia unlikely. Furthermore, the tachycardia is irregular, which makes AVNRT with block to the atrium also unlikely. Atrial activation in the high right atrium precedes the His, which excludes retrograde atrial activation. Junctional bigeminy cannot be excluded, although continuous block to the atrium is unusual.

In this tracing, one sinus beat produces two QRS complexes. Antegrade conduction occurs through both the fast pathway and the slow pathway, which explains the second complex not preceded by the atrium. Ablation of the slow pathway restored singular fast pathway conduction. Patients with a dual response are often not inducible for AVNRT, as the similar refractory periods of the two pathways do not facilitate reentry and, most importantly, retrograde conduction is poor or absent.

Reference

1.   Bradfield J, Buch E, Tung R, Shivkumar K. Recurrent irregular tachycardia that consistently terminates on a P wave. *J Cardiovasc Electrophysiol.* 2012:21(9):1062-1063.

Question

What is the most likely mechanism for this tachycardia induced in a 23-year-old woman?

A) Atrial tachycardia

B) AV node reentry

C) Ventricular tachycardia

D) Orthodromic AV reentry

Figure 3.G.1

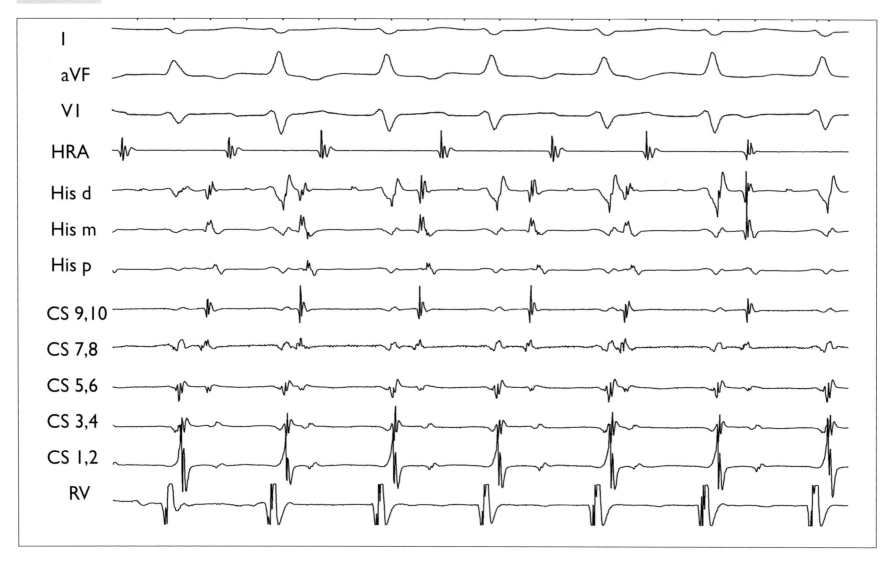

Figure 3.G.2

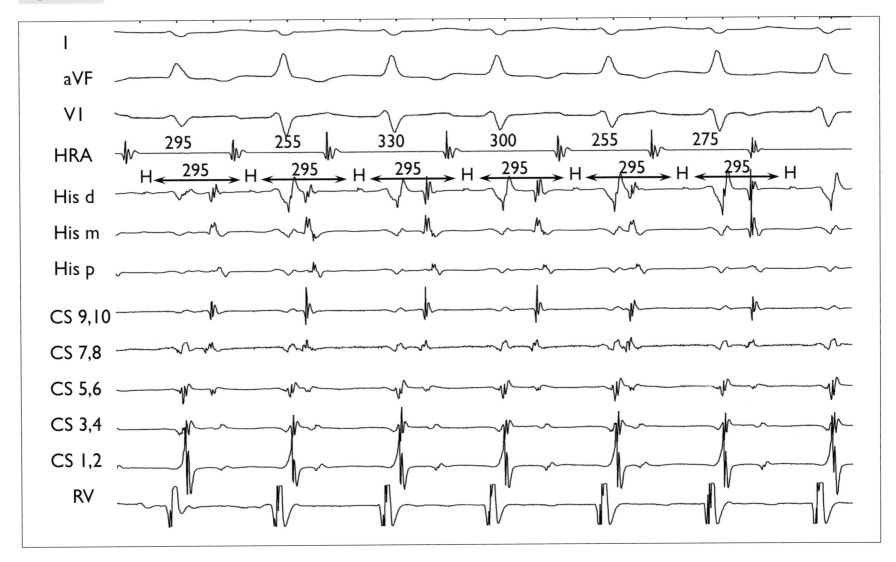

Answer

The correct answer is **B. AVNRT** is seen with variable conduction to the atrium.

When "wobble" or oscillation is seen during tachycardia, it provides an opportunity to distinguish the primary activation that drives subsequent activation. The oscillation in the atrium with variable VA intervals makes retrograde bypass tract conduction unlikely, as VA linking is usually present. With atrial tachycardia, the H-H intervals would be expected to follow the preceding A-A intervals, which is not seen.

In this case, only the H-H interval (295 ms) is constant, which is most consistent with AVNRT. Retrograde atrial activation is earliest in CS 7,8 which is consistent with a left-sided extension of the slow pathway. The oscillation in the retrograde atrial conduction is explained by variable upper common pathway conduction. In addition to the His driving the tachycardia, the narrow-complex morphology with a positive HV interval is not consistent with ventricular tachycardia.

References

1. Crawford TC, Mukerji S, Good E, et al. Utility of atrial and ventricular cycle length variability in determining the mechanism of paroxysmal supraventricular tachycardia. *J Cardiovasc Electrophysiol.* 2007;18(7):698-703.

2. Jongnarangsin K, Pumprueg S, Prasertwitayakij N, et al. Utility of tachycardia cycle length variability in discriminating atrial tachycardia from ventricular tachycardia. *Heart Rhythm.* 2010;7(2):225-228.

Question

What mechanism of tachycardia is demonstrated by this pacing maneuver in a 23-year-old man after slow pathway modification was attempted?

A) AVNRT

B) Atrial tachycardia

C) Junctional tachycardia

D) Ventricular tachycardia

Figure 3.H.1

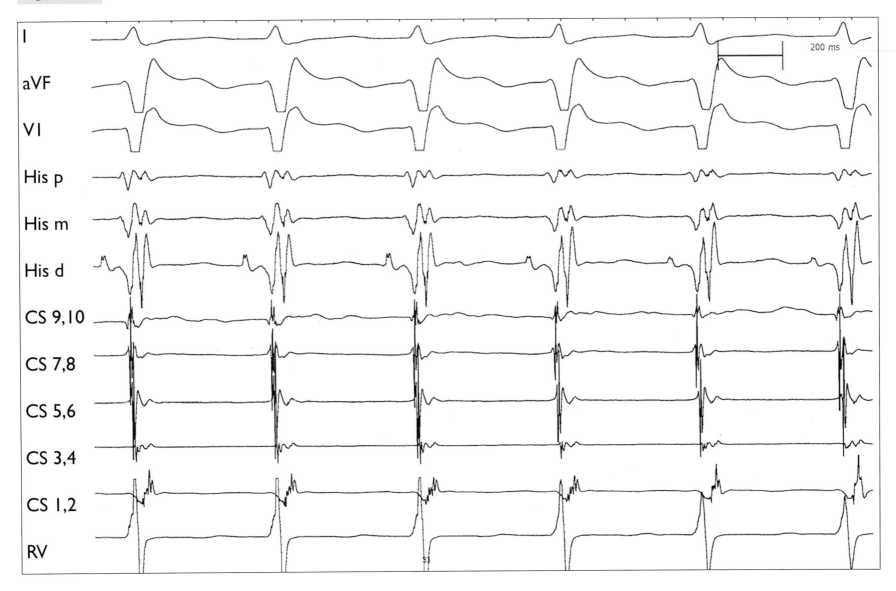

Figure 3.H.2

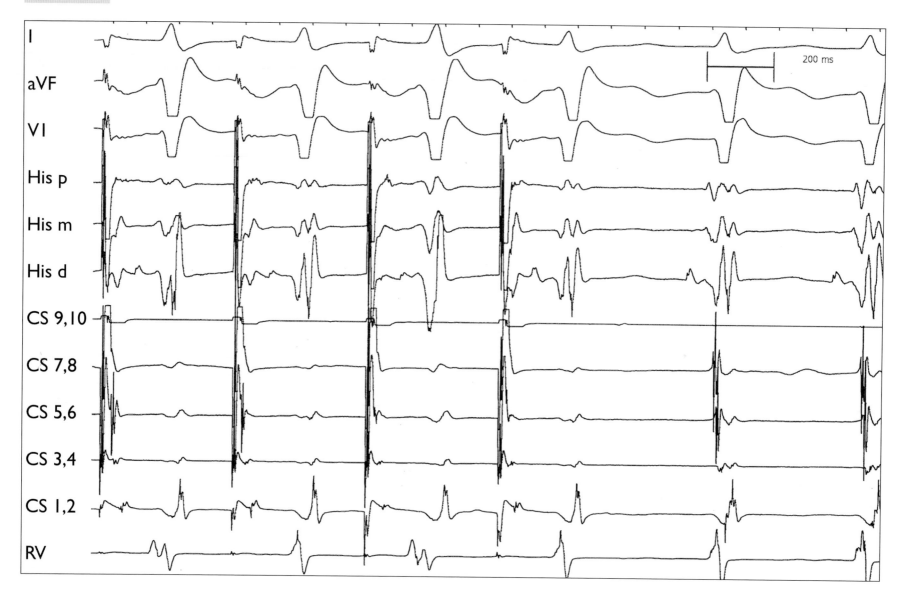

Figure 3.H.3

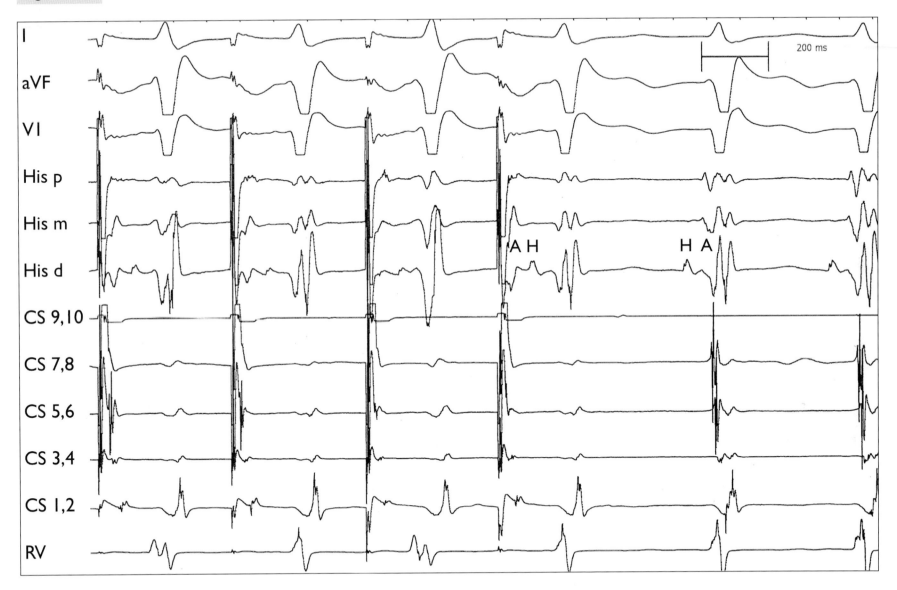

Answer

The correct answer is **C**. **Junctional tachycardia (JT)** is demonstrated with atrial overdrive pacing.

JT can be seen as a result of automaticity during slow pathway modification as well as after it. Differentiation between JT and AVNRT is critical to determine if further ablation is necessary. Atrial overdrive pacing is performed 20–30 ms faster than the tachycardia cycle length until the His is advanced to the paced cycle length. After atrial overdrive pacing, a JT that is transiently suppressed reinitiates with a His, resulting in an A-H-H-A response. AVNRT demonstrates an A-H-A response after atrial overdrive pacing that entrains the His down the slow pathway antegradely.

Atrial tachycardia is excluded as the septal VA time is <70 ms and should not reinitiate with a His electrogram. Ventricular tachycardia typically has a retrograde His and is not expected to have the identical narrow-complex morphology during atrial pacing. For ventricular tachycardia originating from within the conduction system, the HV interval in tachycardia is usually different from the HV during sinus or atrial pacing.

Reference

1. Fan R, Tardos JG, Almasry I, Barbera S, Rashba EJ, Iwai S. Novel use of atrial overdrive pacing to rapidly differentiate junctional tachycardia from atrioventricular nodal reentrant tachycardia. *Heart Rhythm.* 2011;8(6):840-844.

Question

What mechanism of tachycardia is demonstrated in an 18-year-old woman with SVT?

A) AV node reentry

B) Orthodromic reentry

C) Atrial tachycardia

D) Cannot be determined

Figure 3.I.1

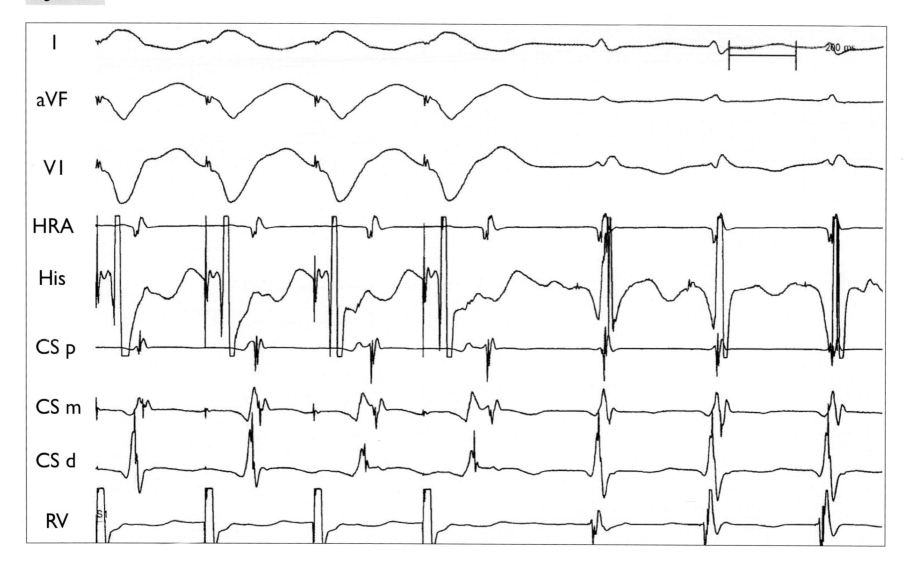

Figure 3.I.2

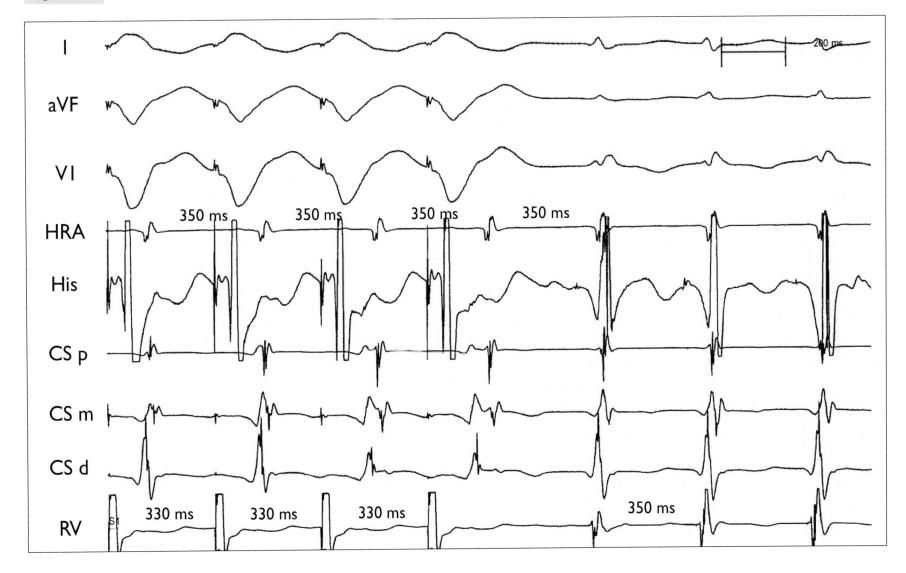

Answer

The correct answer is **D. It cannot be determined**.

A narrow complex tachycardia with a cycle length (CL) of 350 ms after pacing is seen. The right ventricle is paced at 330 ms to entrain the tachycardia. Although ventricular capture is seen, the atrium is not entrained (350 ms). Therefore, the postpacing interval (PPI) and stimulus-to-A interval (SA) cannot be assessed.

However, the tachycardia cannot be orthodromic reentry, since the ventricle is part of the tachycardia circuit and cannot be dissociated from the atrium. Therefore, the differential diagnosis consists of atrial tachycardia and AVNRT with distal block, allowing for dissociation of the tachycardia circuit during pacing.

In such a case, pacing should be repeated at a faster CL and with a longer duration to allow for penetration into the circuit. When the atrium is accelerated to the pacing CL (300 ms), a postpacing V-A-H-V response is seen, which excludes atrial tachycardia (V-A-A-H-V). The PPI–CL is 565 – 330 ms = 235 ms (>110 ms, after correcting for AH decrement) and SA–VA is 175 ms (>85 ms), which is consistent with the diagnosis of AVNRT. The simultaneous ventricular and atrial activation (septal VA <70 ms) is also diagnostic of AVNRT.

References

1. Knight BP, Zivin A, Souza J, et al. A technique for the rapid diagnosis of atrial tachycardia in the electrophysiology laboratory. *J Am Coll Cardiol.* 1999;33(3):775-781.

2. Knight BP, Ebinger M, Oral H, et al. Diagnostic value of tachycardia features and pacing maneuvers during paroxysmal supraventricular tachycardia. *J Am Coll Cardiol.* 2000:36(2):574-582.

Figure 3.I.3

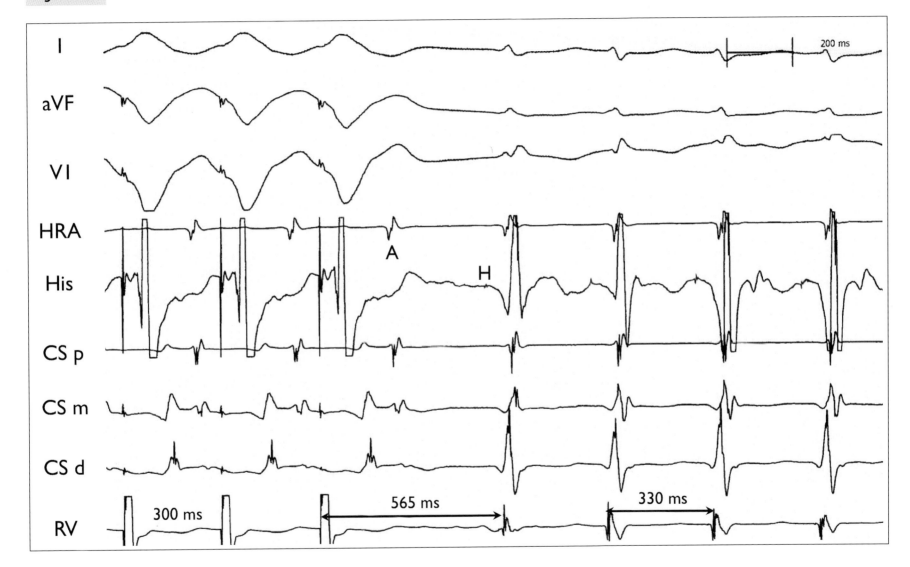

Question

What mechanism of tachycardia is most likely demonstrated after slow pathway modification in an 18-year-old woman?

A) AVNRT

B) Atrial tachycardia

C) Junctional tachycardia

D) Ventricular tachycardia

Figure 3.J.1

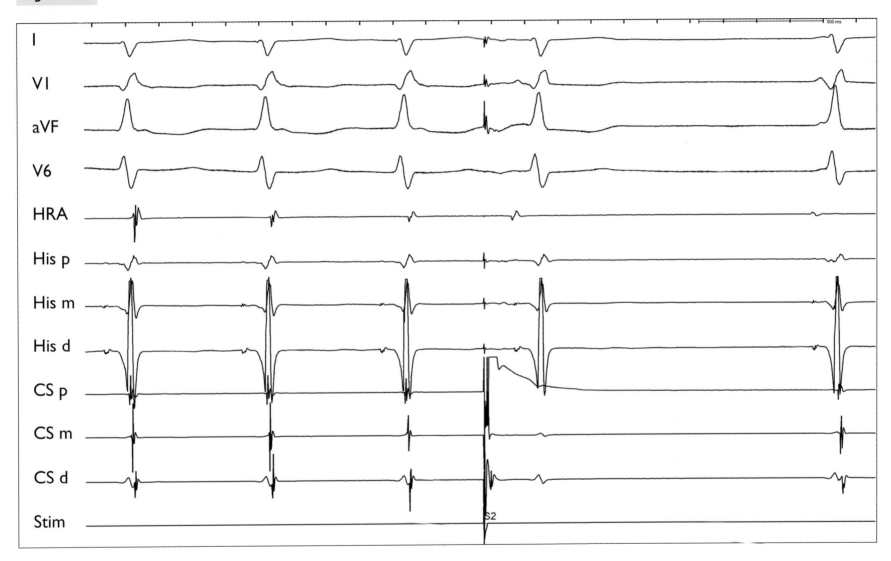

Answer

The correct answer is **A**. **AV nodal reentry tachycardia (AVNRT)** is most likely demonstrated with this pacing maneuver that conceals the fast pathway.

Differentiation between junctional tachycardia (JT) and AVNRT is particularly critical to determine if further ablation is necessary. In this example, ventricular tachycardia is unlikely, as the rhythm is narrow complex. Atrial tachycardia rarely exhibits simultaneous atrial and ventricular activation.

With a premature atrial extrastimulus, the AVNRT can be advanced antegradely down the slow pathway (long AH interval) or terminated if the fast pathway is engaged antegradely, rendering the retrograde limb refractory. JT can be advanced with a short AH interval down the fast pathway, but is not expected to terminate with a single atrial premature stimulus. In this case, the extrastimulus does not advance the subsequent His, which is conducted from the antegrade slow pathway. However, termination of the tachycardia occurs in the retrograde fast pathway, which implies that concealed conduction into the fast pathway occurred antegradely.

Figure 3.J.2

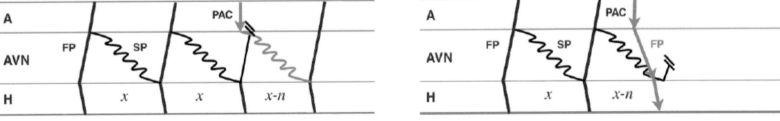

His refractory PAC

JT: collision

AVNRT: advance long AH

Early PAC

JT: advance short AH

AVNRT: advance short AH with termination

Source: Padanilam BJ, Manfredi MD, Steinberg LA, Olson JA, Fogel RI, Prystowsky EN. Differentiating junctional tachycardia and atrioventricular node re-entry tachycardia based on response to atrial extrastimulus pacing. *J Am Coll Cardiol.* 2008;52:1711-1717. With permission from Elsevier.

Reference

1.   Padanilam BJ, Manfredi MD, Steinberg LA, Olson JA, Fogel RI, Prystowsky EN. Differentiating junctional tachycardia and atrioventricular node re-entry tachycardia based on response to atrial extra-stimulus pacing. *J Am Coll Cardiol.* 2008;52:1711-1717.

Question

What is the mechanism of tachycardia in a 45-year-old man with recurrent palpitations?

A) Atrial tachycardia

B) Orthodromic reentry

C) Antidromic reentry

D) AV node reentry

Figure 3.K.1

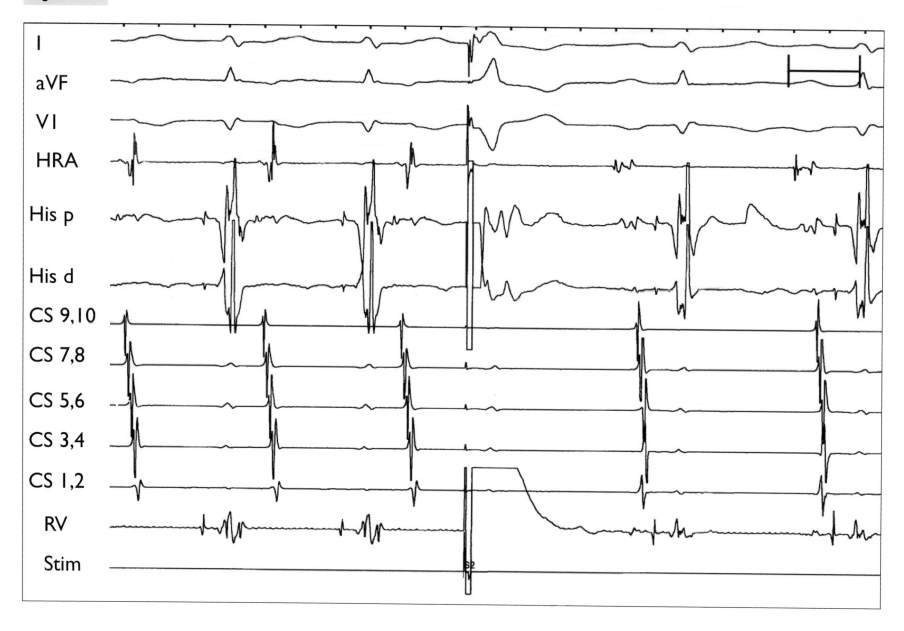

Figure 3.K.2

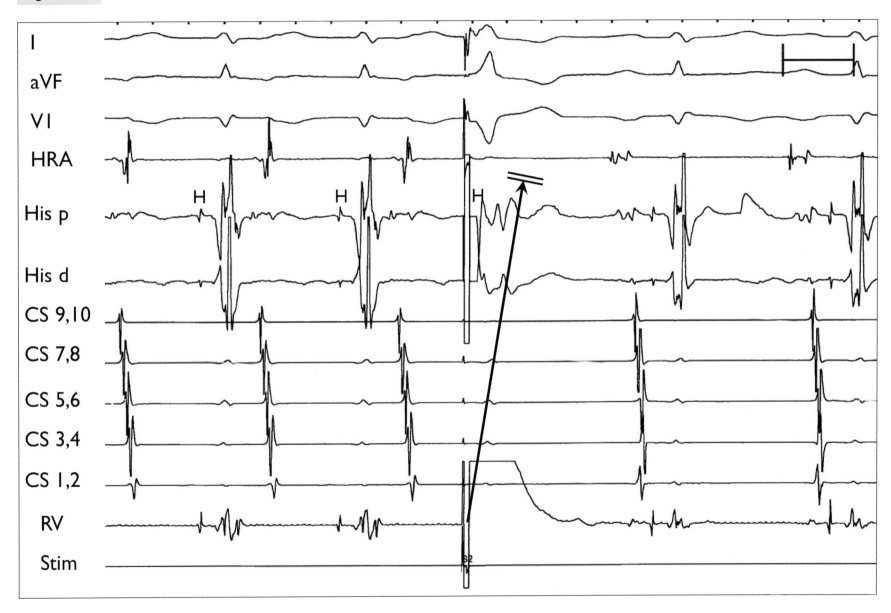

Answer

The correct answer is **B**. **Orthodromic reentrant** tachycardia is proven with termination from a His-refractory PVC.

Antidromic tachycardia is incorrect, as it manifests as a wide-complex tachycardia due to preexcitation. The presence of a bypass tract can be proven with an extranodal response to parahisian pacing and by effecting a change in atrial timing with a His-refractory PVC. PVCs delivered within 50 ms (VH time often exceeds baseline HV interval) of an expected His activation are considered His synchronous. The His bundle is refractory at that time, and retrograde conduction cannot occur via the AV node. When the atrial activation is advanced, or preexcited, a bypass tract is present.

However, the mere presence of a bypass tract does not necessitate participation in tachycardia. Proof of participation in tachycardia requires either (1) delay of the atrial activation, or postexcitation, which is seen with slowly conducting decremental bypass tracts, or (2) termination of the tachycardia without conduction to the atrium. In this case, the PVC is delivered within 40 ms of the next anticipated His depolarization, and tachycardia terminates with block in the parahisian bypass tract. Note that the earliest atrial activation during tachycardia is in the RV channel, which is in a parahisian location.

Reference

1. Knight BP, Ebinger M, Oral H, et al. Diagnostic value of tachycardia features and pacing maneuvers during paroxysmal supraventricular tachycardia. *J Am Coll Cardiol*. 2000;36:574-582.

Question

What is the most likely rhythm recorded in a 70-year-old woman with a 5-year history of palpitations?

A) Atrial tachycardia 2:1 to 1:1

B) Atrial tachycardia 2:1 into AV node reentry

C) Atrial flutter 2:1 into junctional tachycardia

D) AV node reentry 2:1 to 1:1

Figure 3.L.1

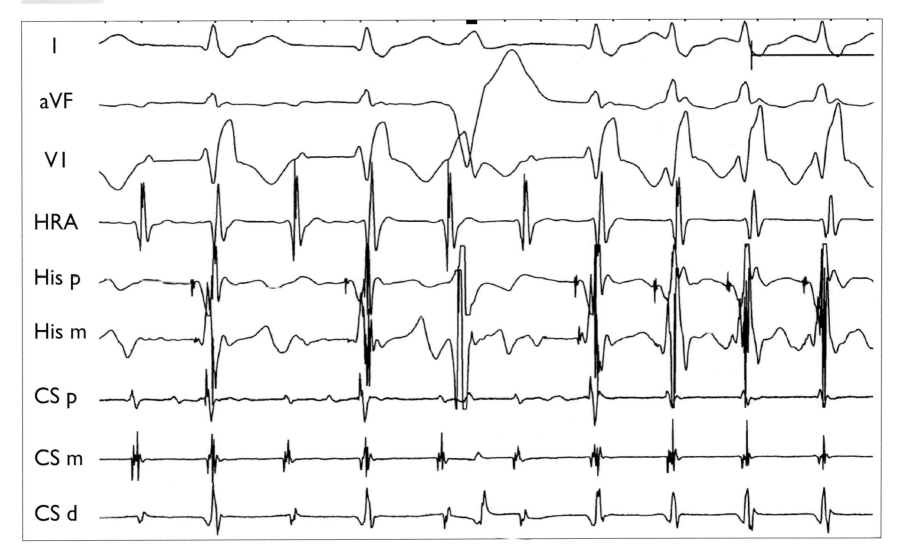

Answer

The correct answer is **D. AV node reentry converts from 2:1 to 1:1** after a PVC.

The initial part of the tracing demonstrates 2:1 conduction to the ventricle with right bundle branch block. Importantly, the atrial rate throughout the tracing is constant (290 ms). Therefore, a change to a different tachycardia mechanism is unlikely. The septal VA time during the conducted beats is <70 ms, which is highly suggestive of AVNRT. During atrial tachycardia, the septal VA time is unlikely to be simultaneous, although conduction with a long PR cannot be completely ruled out. When a P wave is exactly midway between the two QRS complexes, AVNRT with 2:1 block is most likely. Block during AVNRT is commonly seen below the His, but can also occur in the lower common pathway, as seen in this case (absence of His during block).

The PVC likely "peels back" the refractoriness of the AV node and allows for 1:1 conduction to resume. The timing of the PVC occurs during a period of expected block in the lower common pathway. The AV node is rendered refractory for the subsequent beat of AVNRT, allowing for an additional tachycardia cycle length to recover excitability.

Reference

1. Man KC, Brinkman K, Bogun F, et al. 2:1 atrioventricular block during atrioventricular node reentrant tachycardia. *J Am Coll Cardiol.* 1996;28(7):1770-1774.

*Q*uestion

What is the most likely tachycardia mechanism in an 18-year-old man with long-standing palpitations?

A) Junctional tachycardia

B) Atrial tachycardia

C) Orthodromic reentry

D) AV node reentry

Figure 3.M.1

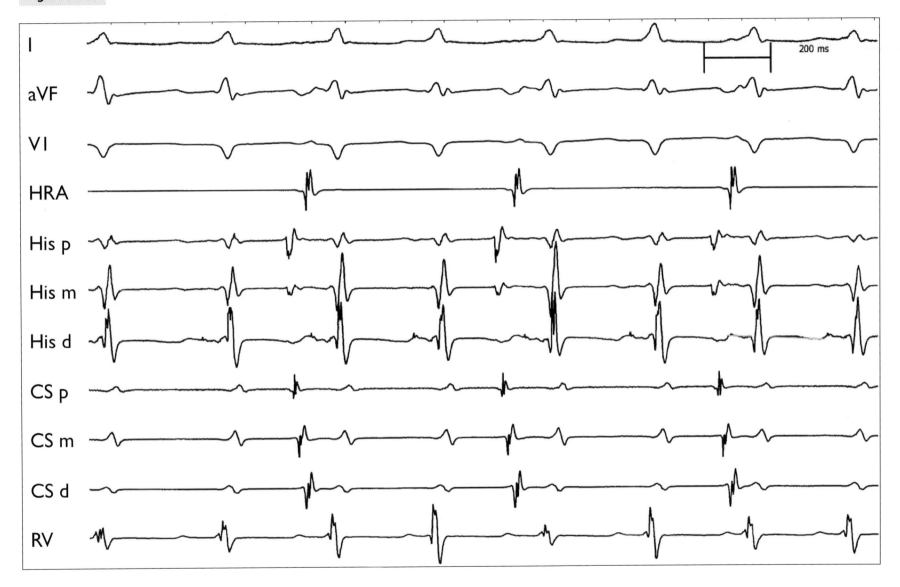

Answer

The correct answer is **A. Junctional tachycardia** is seen in this tracing.

The most important feature is that there are fewer atrial events than ventricular events. Therefore, atrial tachycardia and orthodromic reentry cannot be the mechanism, as the atrium is a necessary component in both. Typical AV node reentry with block to the atrium is a possibility, although retrograde fast pathway activation is typically within 70 ms of septal ventricular activation. Atypical AV node reentry is unlikely, as coronary sinus atrial activation precedes His atrial activation during retrograde slow pathway conduction.

By deduction, junctional tachycardia with retrograde block to the atrium is most likely. A His potential is seen preceding each beat, and slight oscillations in the tachycardia cycle length are predicted by changes in the H-H intervals.

Reference

1. Garson A Jr, Gillette PC. Functional ectopic tachycardia in children: electrocardiography, electrophysiology and pharmacologic response. *Am J Cardiol.* 1979:44:298–302.

Case 3.N

Question

What is the most likely tachycardia mechanism in a
35-year-old woman with palpitations?

A) AV node reentry with aberration

B) Atriofascicular (Mahaim) tachycardia

C) Ventricular tachycardia

D) Bundle branch reentry

Figure 3.N.1

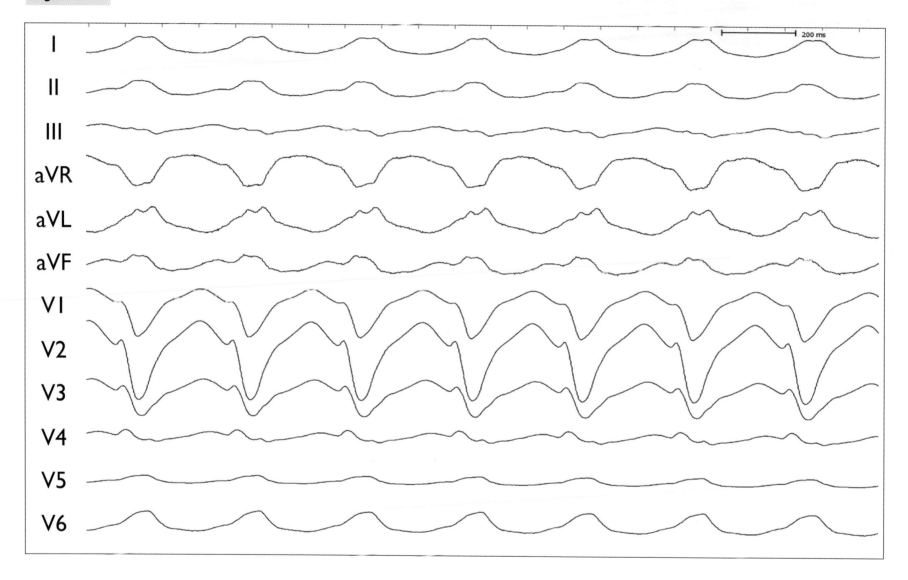

Figure 3.N.2

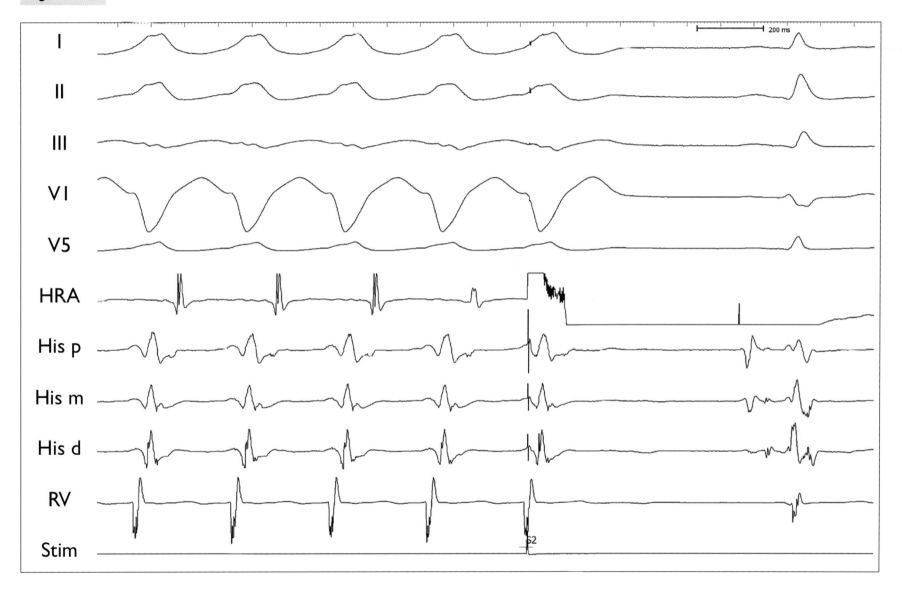

*A*nswer

The correct answer is **B**. A **Mahaim tachycardia** is seen in this tracing.

Although originally described as fasciculoventricular and nodoventricular, Mahaim tachycardias refer to atriofascicular accessory pathways. The resting ECG is usually normal, as these pathways characteristically have decremental antegrade conduction without retrograde conduction. Preexcited Mahaim tachycardias have a left bundle branch block morphology with transition at V_4 or later. During tachycardia, a His potential is not evident, as it occurs within the ventricular electrogram due to preexcitation (negative HV) and the RV is activated at the QRS onset. Supraventricular tachycardia with aberration would have a conducted HV interval, and bundle branch reentry typically has an HV longer than in sinus rhythm.

Termination of the wide-complex tachycardia with a premature single atrial extrastimulus without activation of the ventricle makes ventricular tachycardia unlikely. Much like a His-refractory PVC that terminates a narrow-complex tachycardia without conduction to the atrium, participation of a bypass tract is demonstrated. This is most specific when the PAC is delivered during septal atrial refractoriness, as seen in this case.

References

1. Mahaim I, Bennatt A. Nouvelles recherches sur les connections superieures de la branche du faisceau de His-Tawara avec cloison interventriculaire. *Cardiologia*. 1937;1:61.

2. Tchou P, Lehmann MH, Jazayeri M, Akhtar M. Atriofascicular connection or a nodoventricular Mahaim fiber? Electrophysiologic elucidation of the pathway and associated reentrant circuit. *Circulation*. 1988;77(4):837.

Case 3.0

Question

What is the mechanism of arrhythmia demonstrated by atrial pacing in this 65-year-old man?

A) Atrial tachycardia

B) Antidromic reentry

C) Bundle branch reentry

D) Myocardial ventricular tachycardia

Figure 3.0.1

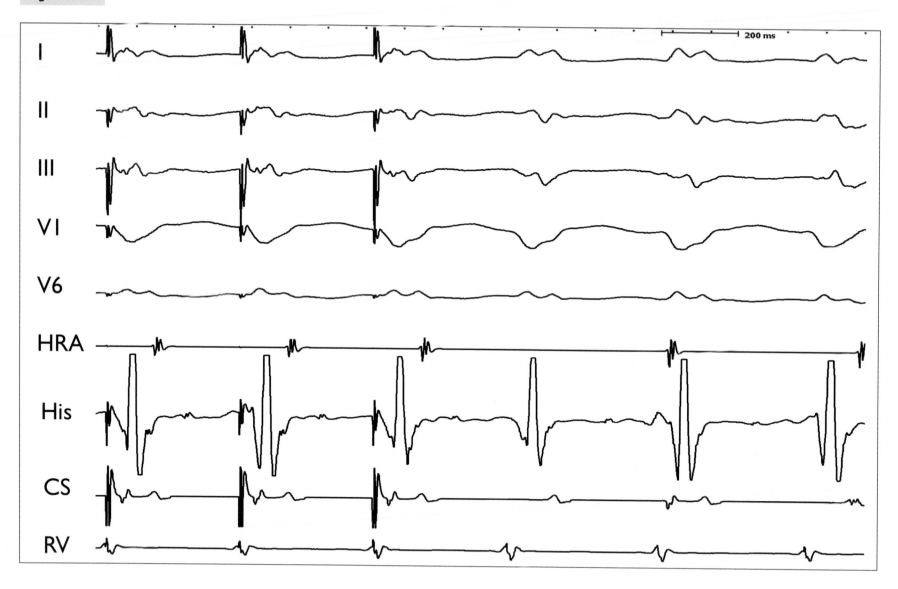

Figure 3.O.2

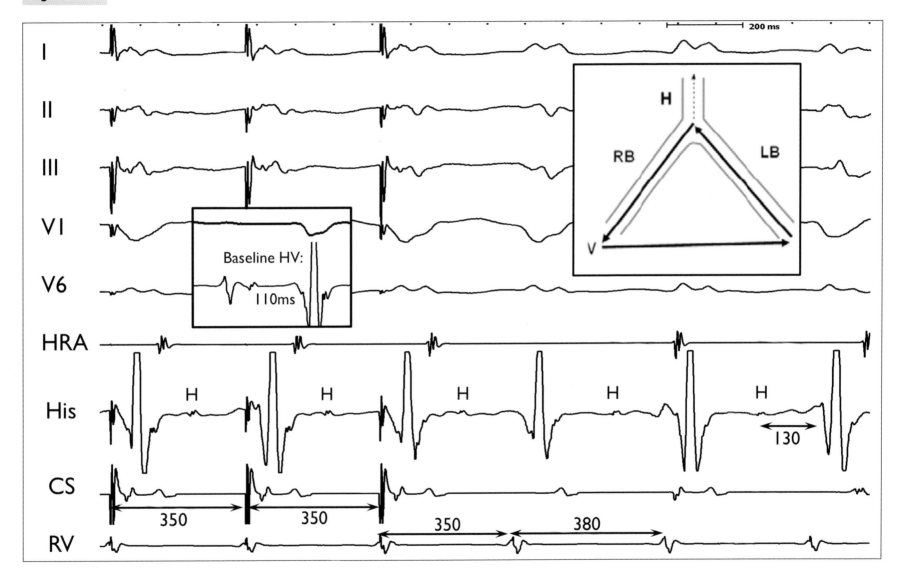

*A*nswer

The correct answer is **C. Bundle branch reentry (BBR)** is demonstrated by atrial entrainment.

A wide-complex tachycardia is seen, and during atrial overdrive pacing, no significant change in QRS morphology is seen. The HV during tachycardia is 130 ms (longer than baseline 110 ms), which is highly suggestive of BBR. Underlying His-Purkinje disease is the rule, and functional conduction delay during tachycardia results in a longer HV interval during BBR. Antidromic tachycardia and myocardial VT typically have negative HV intervals. Importantly, atrioventricular dissociation is seen after entrainment in this tracing, which excludes both atrial tachycardia and antidromic tachycardia.

In BBR with left bundle branch morphology, conduction occurs retrogradely up the left bundle into the His bundle, and antegradely down the right bundle. Concealed entrainment of ventricular tachycardia from the atrium proves involvement of the conduction system. Entrainment from the RV apex, which demonstrates the earliest ventricular activation, shows manifest fusion with a postpacing interval that is within 30 ms of the tachycardia cycle length. In contrast to myocardial VT, oscillations in H-H interval precede and predict V-V changes in BBR.

References

1. Akhtar M, Gilbert C, Wolf FG, Schmidt DH. Reentry within the His-Purkinje system. Elucidation of reentrant circuit using right bundle branch and His bundle recordings. *Circulation.* 1978;58(2):295-330.
2. Lloyd EA, Zipes DP, Heger JJ, Prystowsky EN. Sustained ventricular tachycardia due to bundle branch reentry. *Am Heart J.* 1982;104:1095-1097.

Question

What does this pacing maneuver demonstrate in a 23-year-old woman with sustained palpitations?

A) Proof of pathway presence

B) Proof of pathway participation

C) Proof of pathway absence

D) None of the above

Figure 3.P.1

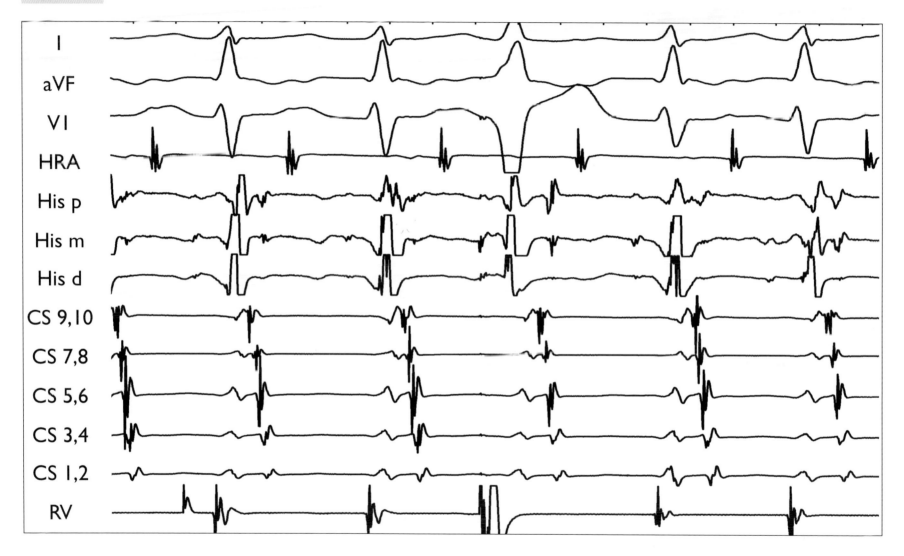

Figure 3.P.2

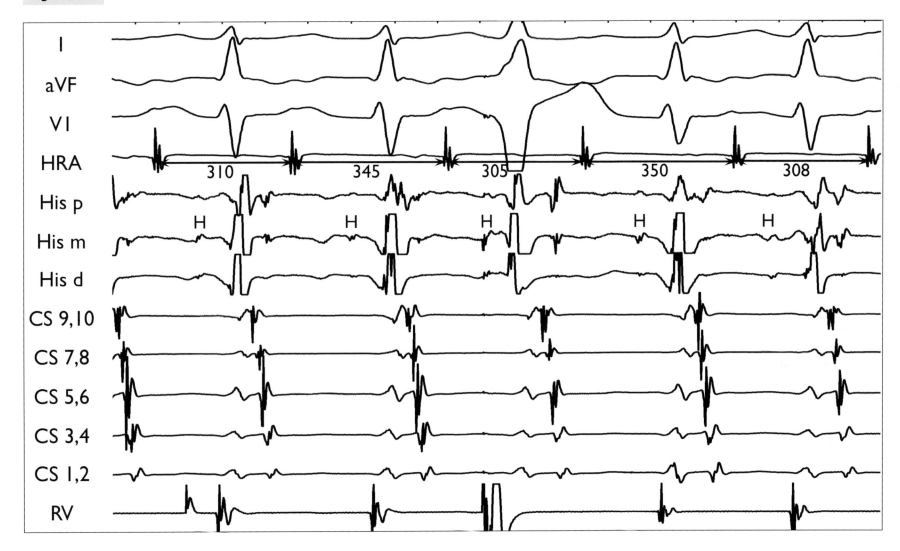

Answer

The correct answer is **D**. The His-refractory PVC is **nondiagnostic**.

The PVC is synchronous with the anticipated His deflection, and the subsequent atrial activation is advanced (305 ms). VA linking is present, and the earliest atrial activation is in the proximal coronary sinus, suggestive of a septal bypass tract. However, close examination of the tachycardia shows significant oscillation or "wobble" of 40 ms, due to variability in the AH interval.

Therefore, the advancement of the atrial activation after the PVC falls on a short sequence of a short–long–short oscillation and cannot be interpreted. Failure to advance the atrium is never definitive proof of accessory pathway absence.

Case 3.Q

Question

Circumferential ablation around the left superior pulmonary vein is performed in a 42-year-old man with paroxysmal atrial fibrillation. What is demonstrated in this tracing?

A) Entrance block

B) Exit block

C) Bidirectional block

D) None of the above

Figure 3.Q.1

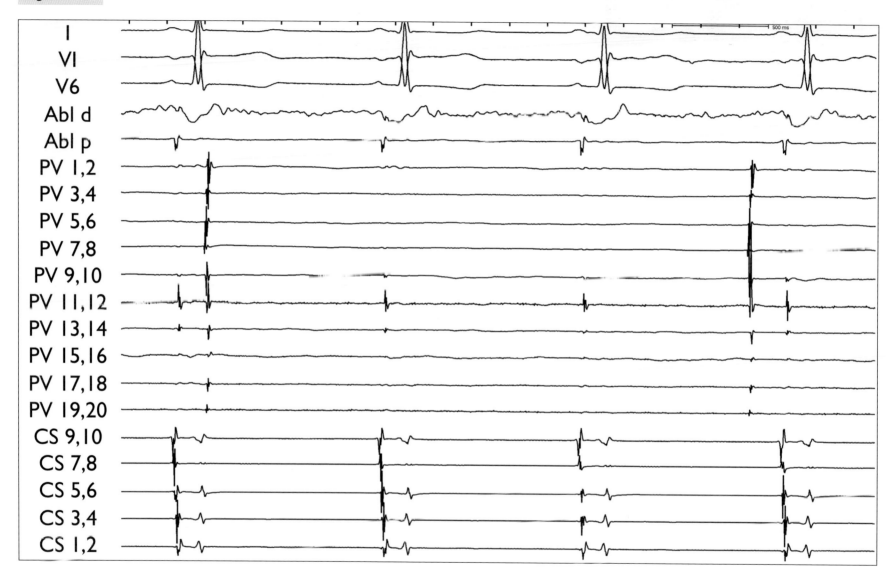

Figure 3.Q.2

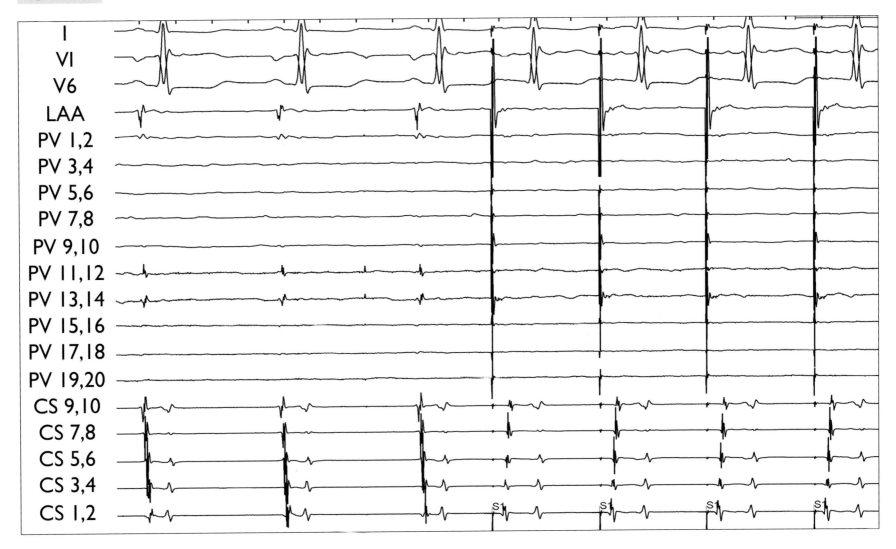

*A*nswer

The correct answer is **B. Exit block** from the pulmonary vein is demonstrated.

The endpoint of pulmonary vein isolation is bidirectional block in and out of the targeted vein. Once the vein is electrically isolated, dissociated pulmonary vein firing that does not result in capture of the left atrium is proof of exit block. In most cases, entrance block is also present when this is seen.

However, demonstration of entrance block requires absence of pulmonary vein potentials seen on the loop catheter placed at the ostium. In this case, persistent pulmonary vein potentials are seen on electrodes 11,12 and 13,14. Pacing from the left atrial appendage results in the disappearance of these potentials, which adequately demonstrates that these signals are far-field from the appendage. After this pacing maneuver, bidirectional block is demonstrated.

References

1. Shah D, Haïssaguerre M, Jaïs P, et al. Left atrial appendage activity masquerading as pulmonary vein potentials. *Circulation*. 2002;105(24):2821-2825.
2. Takahashi Y, O'Neill MD, Jönsson A, et al. How to interpret and identify pulmonary vein recordings with the lasso catheter. *Heart Rhythm*. 2006;3(6):748-750.

Question

What is the most likely diagnosis in this 80-year-old man with presyncope?

A) Atrial tachycardia with aberration

B) AV node reentry with aberration

C) Ventricular tachycardia

D) Orthodromic reentry with aberration

Figure 3.R.1

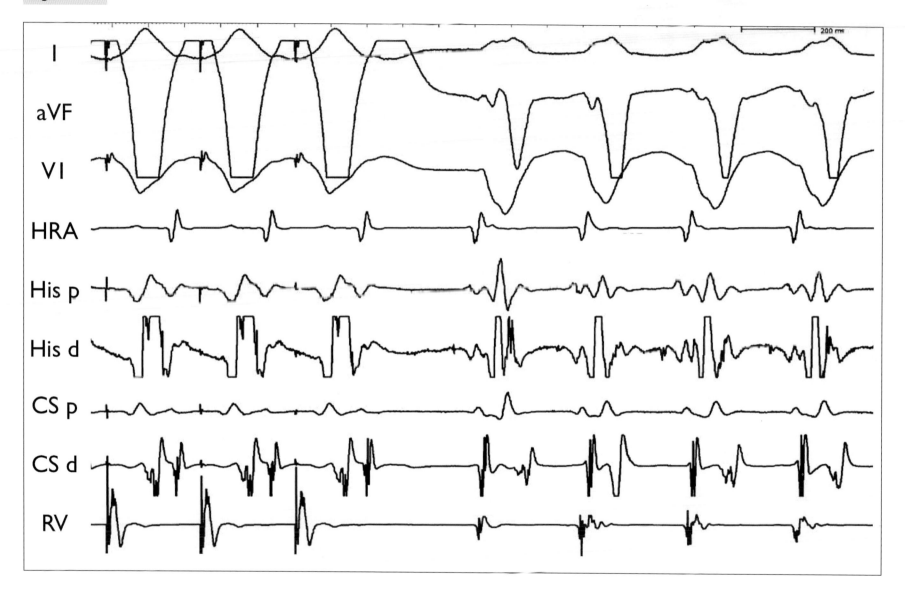

Figure 3.R.2

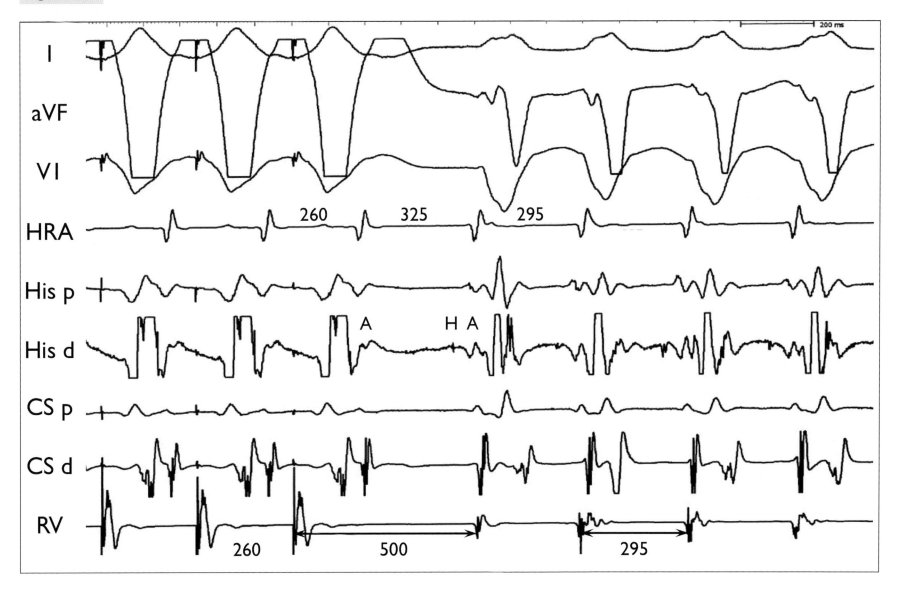

*A*nswer

The correct answer is **B**. This arrhythmia is most consistent with **AV node reentry with left bundle branch block aberration**.

°A prolongation in antegrade AV node conduction is seen after entrainment, and the postpacing interval should be corrected for AH decrement (delta AH − 30 ms). After correction, the PPI-TCL difference (500 − 295 − 30 = 175 ms) is still consistent with AV node reentry (>115 ms).

References

1. Vijayaraman P, Lee BP, Kalahasty G, Wood MA, Ellenbogen KA. Reanalysis of the "pseudo A-A-V" response to ventricular entrainment of supraventricular tachycardia: importance of His-bundle timing. *J Cardiovasc Electrophysiol.* 2006;17(1):25-28.

2. Gonzalez-Torrecilla E, Arenal A, Atienza F, et al. First postpacing interval after tachycardia entrainment with correction for atrioventricular node delay: a simple maneuver for differential diagnosis of atrioventricular nodal reentrant tachycardias versus orthodromic reciprocating tachycardias. *Heart Rhythm.* 2006;3(6):674-679.

Question

Wide-complex tachycardia was induced in a 24-year-old man. What does this pacing maneuver demonstrate?

A) Bystander accessory pathway

B) Presence of pathway with participation in tachycardia

C) Supraventricular tachycardia with left bundle branch aberration

D) Ventricular tachycardia

Figure 3.S.1

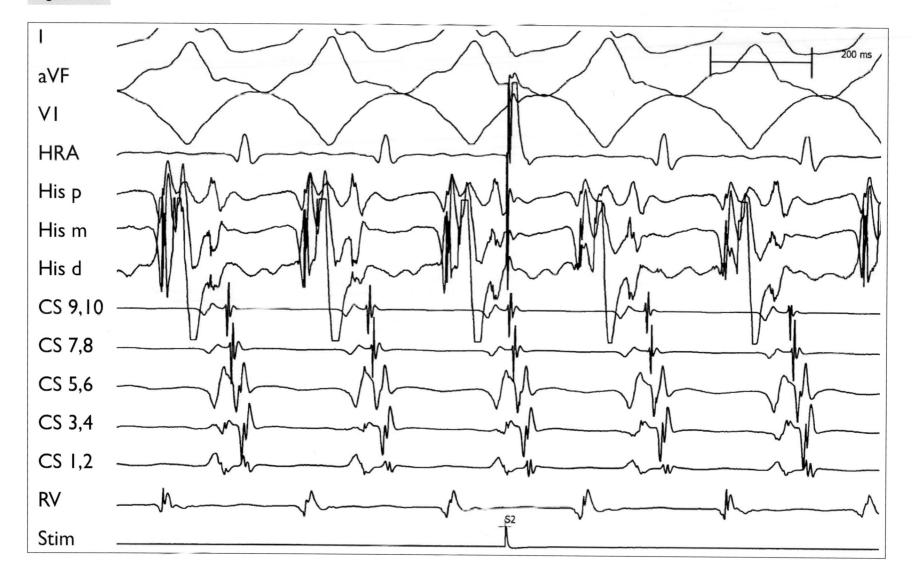

Figure 3.S.2

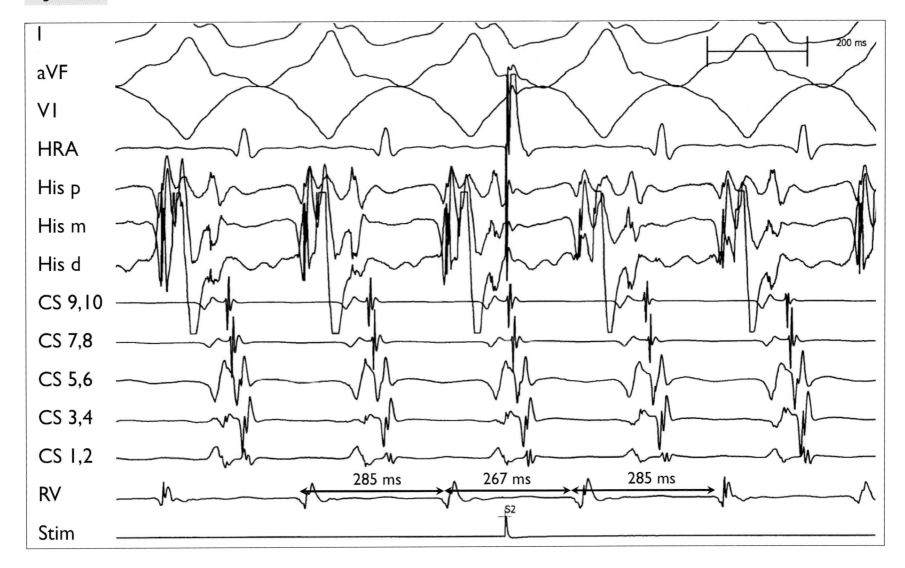

*A*nswer

The correct answer is **B**. This is an **antidromic tachycardia**.

This is a wide-complex tachycardia with no apparent His bundle recording preceding the QRS complexes. Therefore, SVT with aberration is excluded. An atrial extrastimulus given at the time of refractoriness of the His (septal) bundle atrial activation can help determine whether the atrium is part of the circuit, ruling out ventricular tachycardia. This is analogous to His-refractory PVCs delivered during a narrow-complex tachycardia. In this case, the PAC is introduced just after the septal A activation, which implies that any effect on the ventricular is via an accessory pathway.

The right atrial PAC advances the ventricle by 18 ms, proving the presence of the accessory pathway. The tachycardia is reset by the same interval, indicating that the antegrade conduction over the right-sided accessory pathway is an integral part of the circuit and not a bystander pathway. Ventricular tachycardia cannot be reset from the atrium with the same morphology unless it involves the conduction system (positive HV in bundle branch reentry).

References

1. Josephson ME. *Clinical Cardiac Electrophysiology: Techniques and Interpretations*, 4th ed. Philadelphia: Lippincott, Williams & Wilkins, 2008:378.

2. Bardy GH, Packer DL, German LD, Gallagher JJ. Preexcited reciprocating tachycardia in patients with Wolff-Parkinson-White syndrome: incidence and mechanisms. *Circulation*. 1984;70:377-391.

Question

What is demonstrated with the circular loop catheter placed in the right superior pulmonary vein in a 72-year-old man during ablation?

A) Entrance block

B) Exit block

C) Bidirectional block

D) Partial isolation

Figure 3.T.1

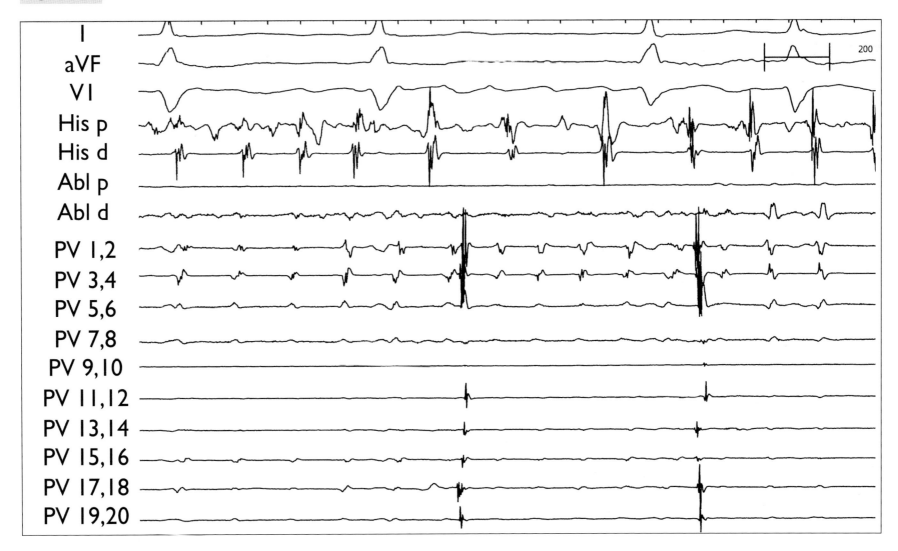

*A*nswer

The correct answer is **A**. Only **entrance block** into the pulmonary vein (PV) can be confirmed.

The rhythm is atrial fibrillation. Low-amplitude, low-frequency potentials are seen on circular bipoles 5–8 and 15–20, consistent with far-field activity. The source of the electrograms recorded in bipoles 1–4 is unclear and appears to indicate fibrillation around these portions of the circular catheter, which would imply conduction into the vein. The position of the catheter should always be confirmed, since part of it may extend beyond the ablation line, giving a false impression of conduction in the antrum.

Isolated, sharp electrograms consistent with PV potentials are noted on the circular loop catheter; these potentials are dissociated from ongoing atrial fibrillation. If conduction into the PV were intact, the faster atrial fibrillatory activity would drive the pulmonary potentials at a more rapid rate. Therefore, entrance block into the vein is present. Exit block cannot be proven during atrial fibrillation. It is possible to partially isolate the vein such that some fascicles may be electrically isolated, giving rise to isolated PV potentials. Therefore, bidirectional block should be checked by pacing maneuvers during sinus rhythm.

Reference

1. Takahashi Y, O'Neill MD, Jönsson A, et al. How to interpret and identify pulmonary vein recordings with the lasso catheter. *Heart Rhythm.* 2006;3(6):748-750.

Question

What does this entrainment response demonstrate in a 65-year-old man with a history of anteroseptal infarction?

A) Remote bystander

B) Outer loop

C) Isthmus

D) Dead-end bystander

Figure 3.U.1

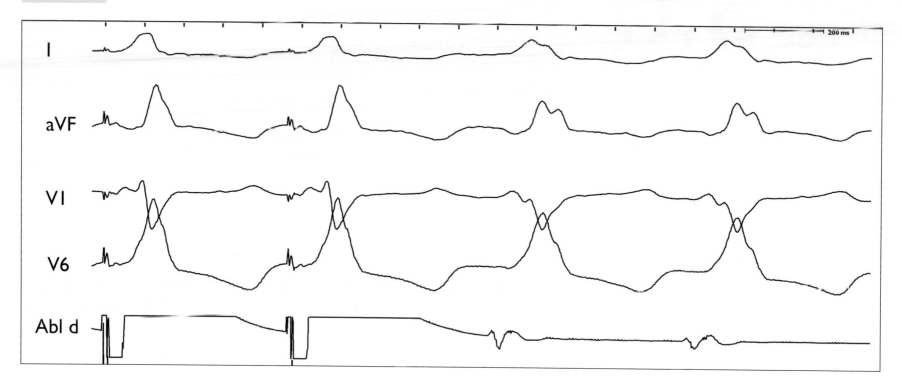

Figure 3.U.2

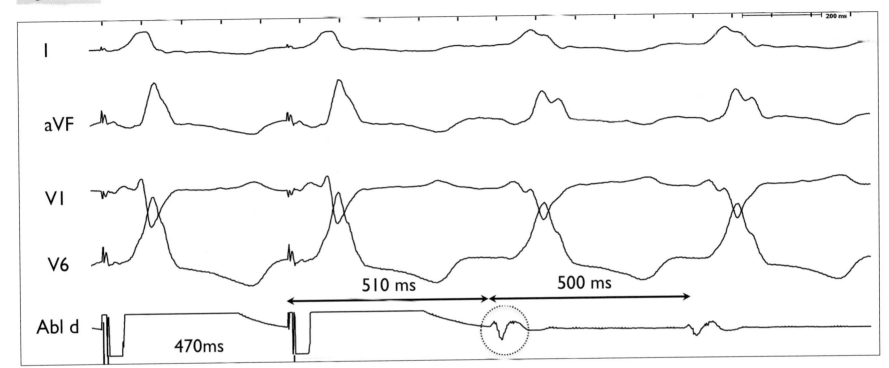

*A*nswer

The correct answer is **B**. This demonstrates entrainment from an **outer loop** site.

Overt, or manifest, fusion is seen on the surface leads during pacing 30 ms faster than the tachycardia cycle length (TCL). Isthmus and dead-end bystander sites exhibit concealed fusion as antidromic wavefront collision occurs within the circuit. At an outer loop site, the antidromic wavefront is not bound within the protected scar channel, resulting in myocardial capture spatially distinct from the circuit exit site.

The postpacing interval (510 ms) is within 30 ms of the TCL (500 ms), indicating that the site is in the circuit. The short EGM-QRS interval indicates proximity toward the exit site. Remote bystanders are spatially distant from the reentrant circuit and exhibit long postpacing intervals and manifest fusion.

Figure 3.U.3

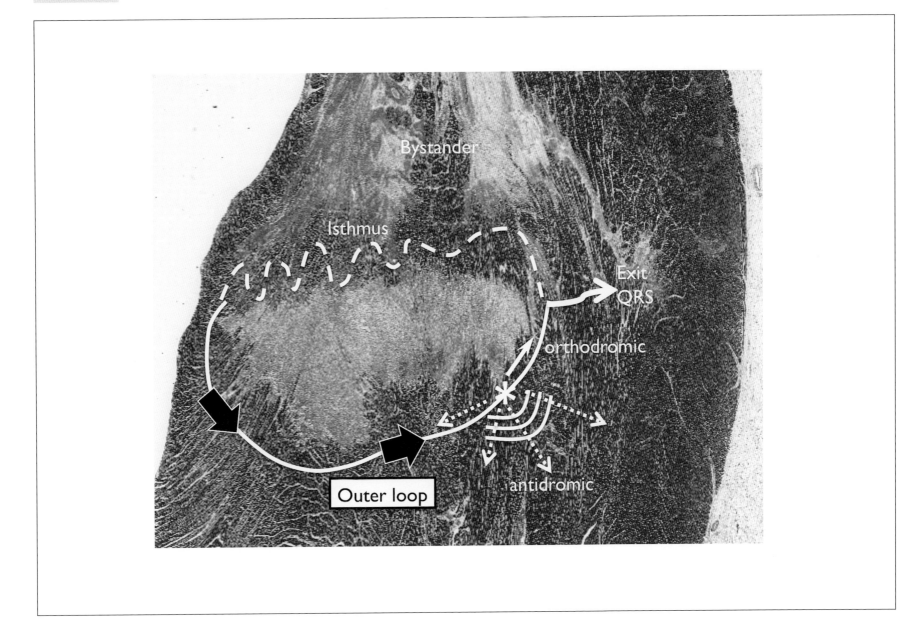

Reference

1. Stevenson WG, Khan H, Sager P, et al. Identification of reentry circuit sites during catheter mapping and radiofrequency ablation of ventricular tachycardia late after myocardial infarction. *Circulation*. 1993;88:1647–1670.

Question

What is the mechanism of tachycardia induced in a 32-year-old female?

A) AV node reentry

B) Orthodromic reentry

C) Atrial tachycardia

D) Junctional tachycardia

Figure 3.V.1

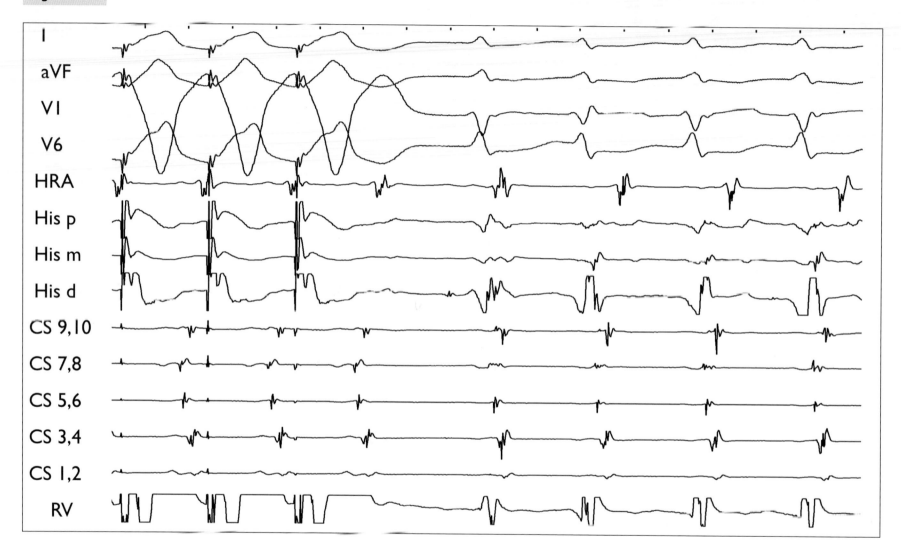

Figure 3.V.2

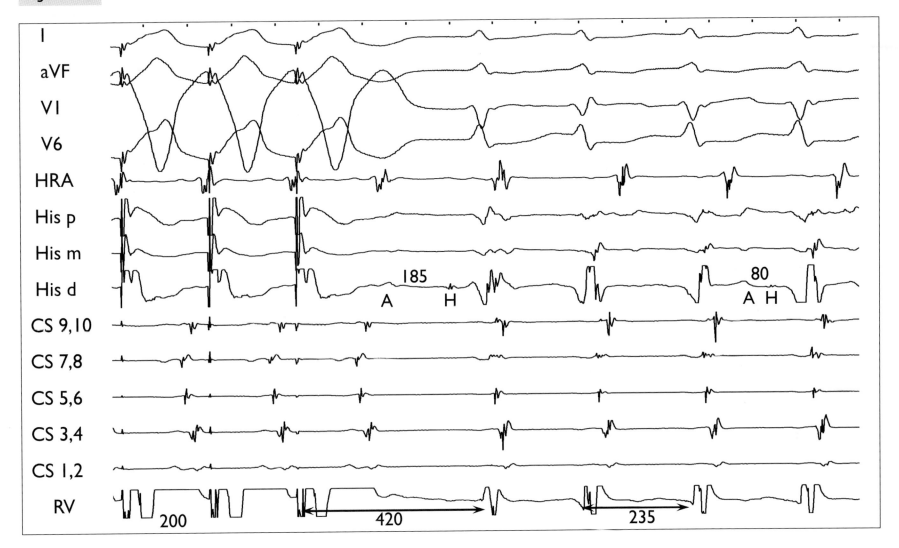

*A*nswer

The correct answer is **C**. This response after ventricular overdrive pacing during orthodromic reentry demonstrates a **long post-pacing interval due to AH delay.**

The earliest atrial activation in CS 7,8 is not typical for slow–fast AVNRT or junctional tachycardia, and the V–A–V response excludes atrial tachycardia. A postpacing interval–tachycardia cycle length difference of >115 ms has been shown to be specific for AV nodal reentry, as the ventricle is not part of the circuit. However, the decrement in the AV node due to accelerating the atrium to the pacing cycle length prolongs the postpacing interval. Therefore, this postpacing AH interval difference from baseline AH (185 − 80 = 105 ms) must be subtracted from the PPI-TCL difference (185 ms) to correct the PPI-TCL difference (80 ms), which is intended to determine the distance of the ventricle from the reentrant circuit. The corrected PPI is <110 ms, which is consistent with orthodromic reentrant tachycardia. The atrial activation in the first beat after entrainment represents fusion of sinus and retrograde left posteroseptal bypass tract.

References

1. Michaud GF, Tada H, Chough S, et al. Differentiation of atypical atrioventricular node re-entrant tachycardia from orthodromic reciprocation tachycardia using a septal accessory pathway by the response to ventricular pacing. *J Am Coll Cardiol.* 2012;38(4):1163–1167.

2. Gonzalez-Torrecilla E, Arenal A, Atienza F, et al. First postpacing interval after tachycardia entrainment with correction for atrioventricular node delay: a simple maneuver for differential diagnosis of atrioventricular nodal reentrant tachycardias versus orthodromic reciprocating tachycardias. *Heart Rhythm.* 2006;3(6):674–679.

Question

What is the diagnosis in a 40-year-old woman with episodic palpitations?

A) Typical AV node reentry

B) Atrial tachycardia

C) Orthodromic reentry

D) Atypical AV node reentry

Figure 3.W.1

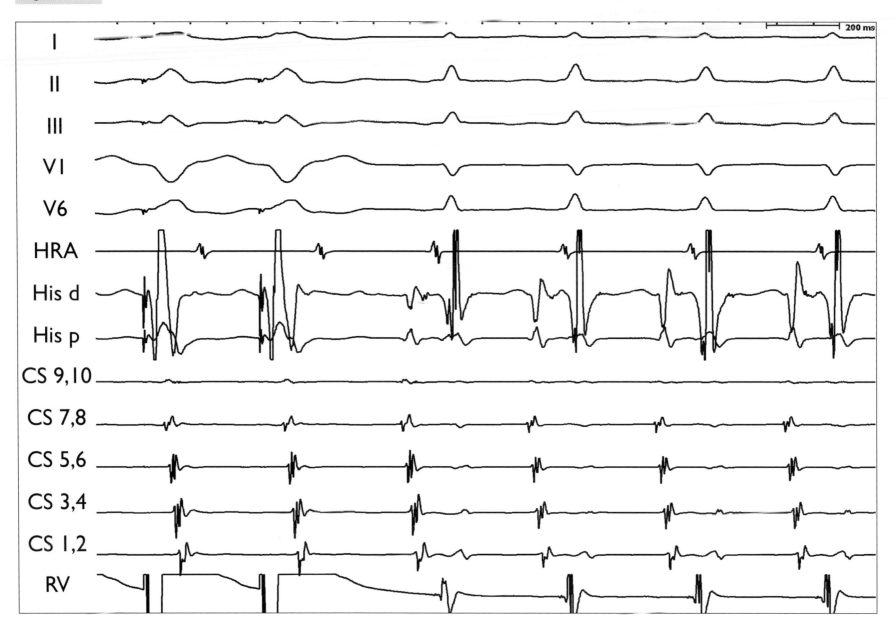

Figure 3.W.2

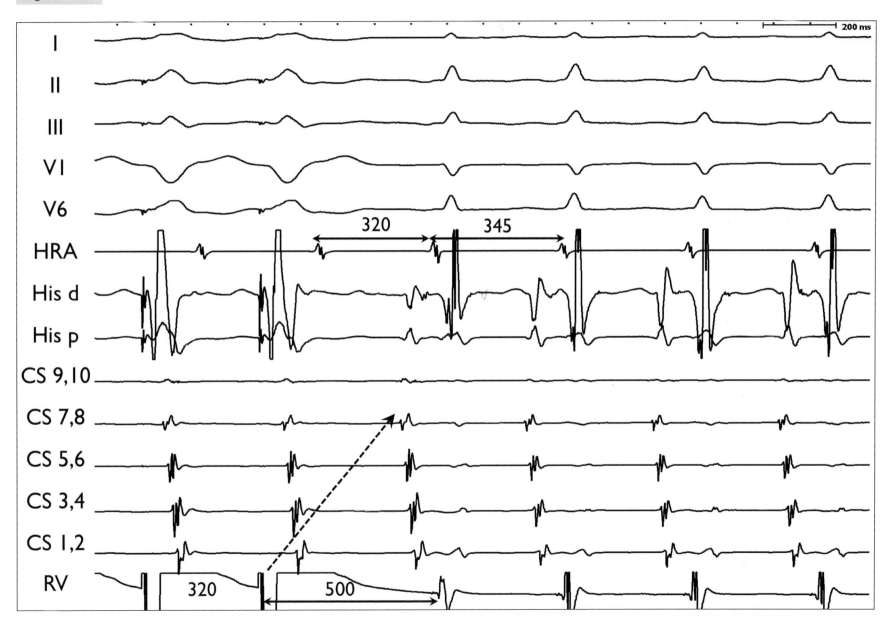

*A*nswer

The correct answer is **D. Atypical AV node reentry** is demonstrated by entrainment.

After the tachycardia is accelerated to the pacing cycle length, a V-A-A-V response is seen. However, the atrium is entrained with a long VA time, with the second atrial event resulting from the last paced ventricular beat (A-A interval 320 ms). This V-A-V response can be misinterpreted for atrial tachycardia, as it is called a "pseudo-V-A-A-V" response. The short AH interval upon cessation of pacing also makes atrial tachycardia unlikely, as it appears to be too rapid to conduct to the His.

The atrial activation is earliest in the proximal coronary sinus, which is consistent with atypical AVNRT. Typical AVNRT frequently has simultaneous atrial and ventricular activation with the earliest atrial activation in the His channel. The postpacing interval-tachycardia cycle length difference of 180 ms (>115 ms) makes orthodromic tachycardia unlikely.

Reference

1. Knight BP, Zivin A, Souza J, et al. A technique for the rapid diagnosis of atrial tachycardia in the electrophysiology laboratory. *J Am Coll Cardiol.* 1999;33(3):775-781.

Case **3.X**

Question

What is the most likely diagnosis in a 31-year-old man with a history of recurrent episodic palpitations?

A) Dual AV node physiology

B) Orthodromic reentry utilizing a left lateral accessory pathway

C) Atrial tachycardia

D) Multiple accessory pathways

Figure 3.X.1

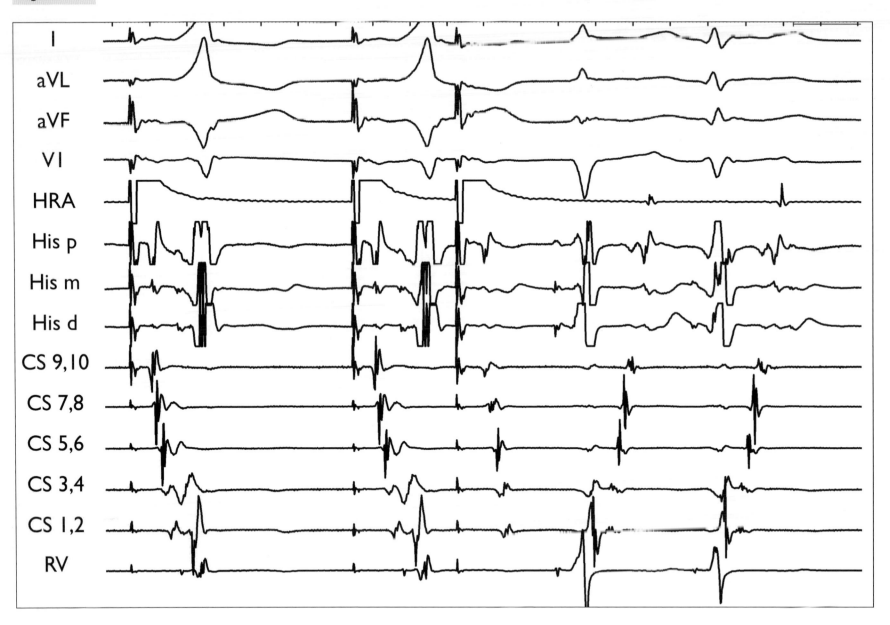

Figure 3.X.2

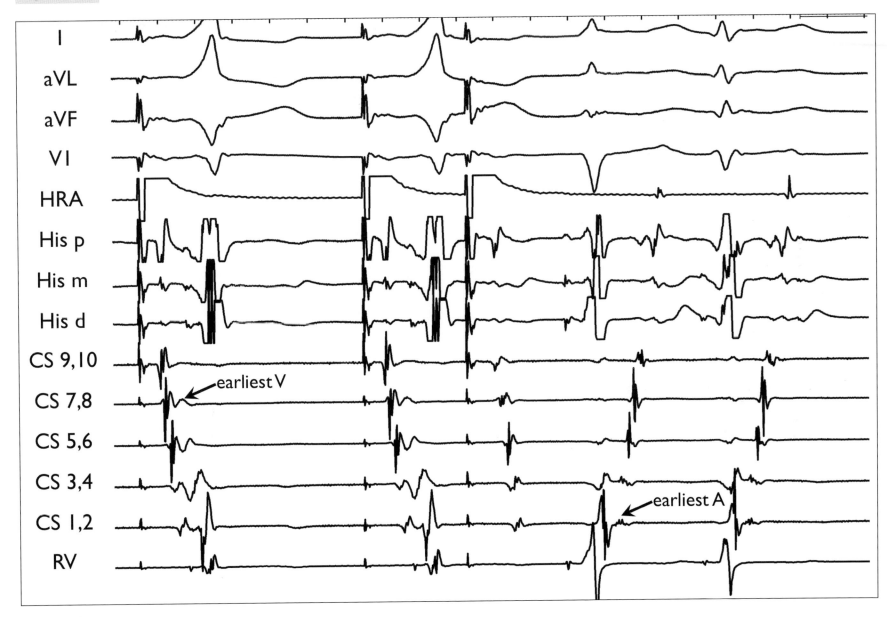

Answer

The correct answer is **D**. **Multiple accessory pathways** are present.

Preexcitation is seen during the atrial pacing train, and the pathway effective refractory period is reached with the extra-stimulus. The preexcitation pattern is not consistent with a left lateral pathway, as the delta waves are positive in leads I and aVL. However, two echo beats utilizing a concealed left lateral pathway occur after the extrastimulus, with CS 1,2 representing the earliest atrial activation. The earliest local ventricular activation of the preexcited complexes is in the proximal coronary sinus, consistent with a left posteroseptal pathway. Although accessory pathways may have an oblique course, the presence of two distinct path-ways is most likely. Pacing from both medial and lateral to the pathway did not show evidence of slanted fiber orientation.

Dual AV node physiology is likely present, as the AH is long prior to the echo beats, although a jump cannot be proven due to antegrade accessory pathway conduction. A left atrial tachycardia is unlikely to be reproducibly initiated with a critical AH interval delay.

Reference

1. Jackman WM, Friday KJ, Yeung-Lai-Wa JA, et al. New catheter technique for recording left free-wall accessory atrioventricular pathway activation. Identification of fiber orientation. *Circulation*. 1998;78(3):598-611.

Question

What does this pacing maneuver demonstrate in a 25-year-old woman with recurrent tachycardia?

A) AV node reentry

B) Atrial tachycardia

C) Accessory pathway presence only

D) Accessory pathway participation

Figure 3.Y.1

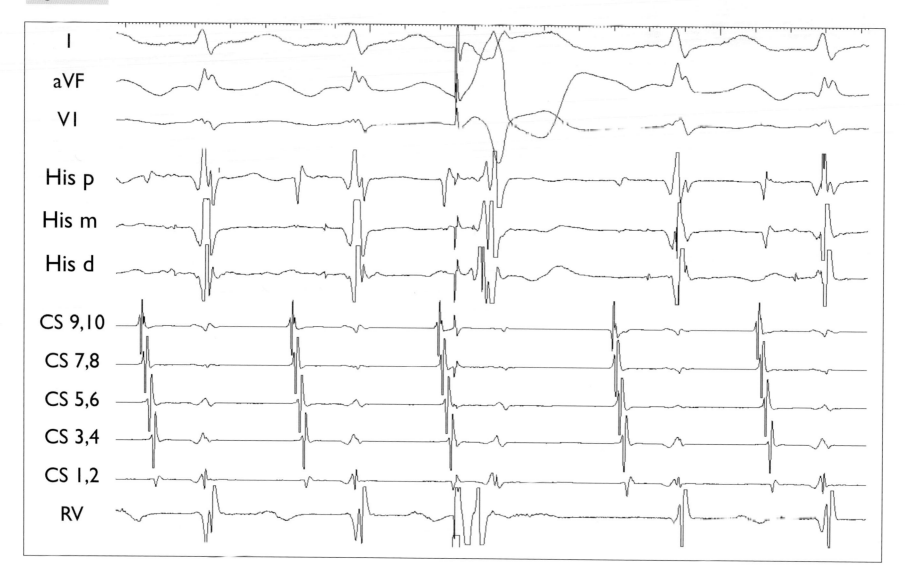

Figure 3.Y.2

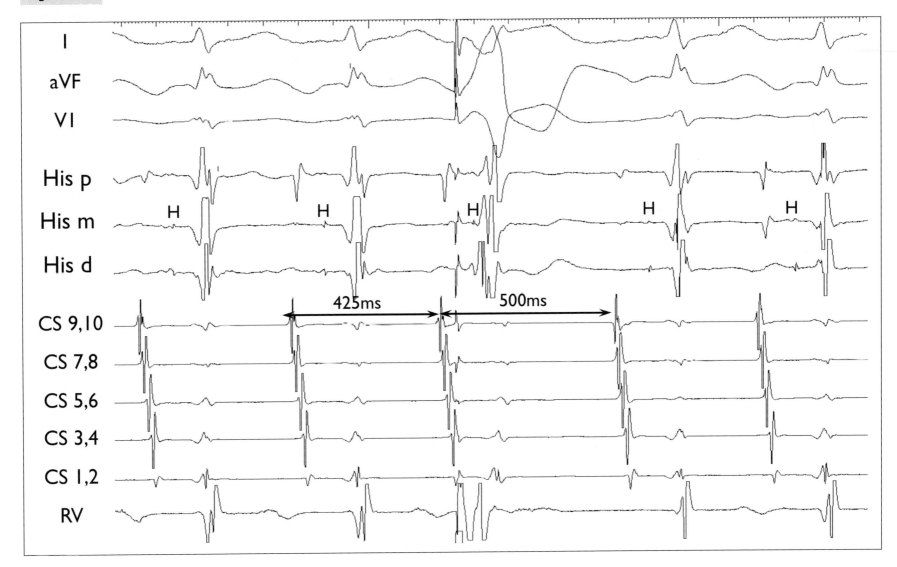

Answer

The correct answer is **D. Presence and participation of an accessory pathway** is demonstrated.

A long RP tachycardia is seen in this tracing with inverted inferior P waves. All mechanisms of SVT are possible, but the change in atrial activation timing after a His-refractory PVC proves that an accessory pathway is present. Because retrograde ventricle-to-His activation timing is usually slower than antegrade HV conduction, a PVC can be delivered at an HV interval prior to the anticipated His and still encounter His refractoriness.

Advancement of the atrial activation with a His-refractory PVC only proves the presence of an accessory pathway, whereas delay, or postexcitation, of the atrial activation proves pathway participation. This is commonly seen in decrementally conducting pathways such as permanent reciprocating junctional tachycardia, with the earliest atrial activation at the coronary sinus ostium. The most extreme form of delay in a decremental pathway is seen when conduction block occurs and tachycardia terminates without atrial activation, which also proves pathway participation.

Reference

1. Chien WW, Cohen TJ, Lee MA, et al. Electrophysiological findings and long-term follow-up of patients with the permanent form of junctional reciprocating tachycardia treated by catheter ablation. *Circulation*. 1992;85(4):1329-1336.

PART 4

Device Tracings

Case 4.A

Background

A 48-year-old male with a past medical history of nonischemic cardiomyopathy, EF 20%, hypertension, paroxysmal atrial fibrillation, and NYHA Class II CHF is evaluated for a shock. The Cameron Subcutaneous ICD was implanted for secondary prevention (spontaneous sustained ventricular tachycardia and structural heart disease). The patient's medical history is also significant for morbid obesity, weighing 508 lbs.

Table 4.A.1 Programmed Parameters	
Shock Zone	200 bpm
Conditional Zone	170 bpm
Therapy	80 J *Reversed*
Sensing Configuration	Alternate Vector
Postshock Pacing	On

The following episode was stored by the SICD while the patient remained hospitalized (Figure 4.A.1).

Question

Which of the following best describes the SICD therapy for this patient?

A) Undersensing VF

B) Oversensing

C) Double detection algorithm

D) Appropriate time to therapy

E) All of the above

Figure 4.A.1

Stored EGM, part 1.

Implant Date: 03/07/2011

Device Settings
Therapy: ON
Shock Zone: 200 bpm
Conditional Shock Zone: 170 bpm
Post Shock Pacing: ON

Gain Setting: 1X
Sensing Configuration: Alternate

S = Sense
P = Pace
N = Noise
T = Tachy Detection
C = Charge Start
. = Discard
⚡ = Shock
🔱 = Episode End

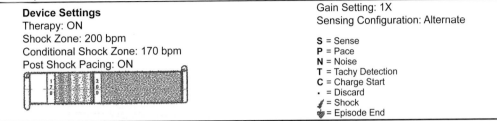

TREATED EPISODE 001: 03/12/2-11 11:28:37 AM   25 mm/sec 2.5 mm/mV
SHOCK IMPEDANCE = 66 ohms FINAL SHOCK POLARITY = REV

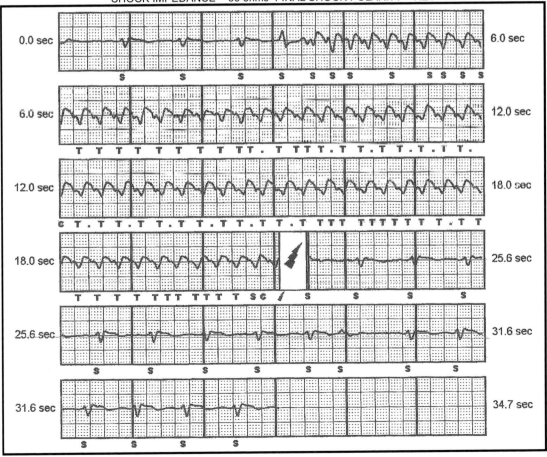

Answer

The correct answer is **E, all of the above**.

In the certification phase, the SICD uses three algorithms to minimize oversensing. These include a template-matching, wide-complex and alternating interval algorithms. These assist with appropriately sensing cardiac events and prevent inappropriate detection due to oversensing T waves and double detection from wide-complex tachycardias. When an interval is discarded due to double detection, the interval is noted with a "." marker, as noted on this stored episode. If a double detection interval is noted, the device will decrement the X/Y counter.

The SICD utilizes the X/Y detection criteria. Once 18 of 24 fast intervals are noted, initial criteria are met. *Persistence* is then used to ensure that the patient remains in a sustained tachycardia prior to charge; the nominal value is two intervals. If two additional tachycardia, "T," events are noted, tachycardia detection is met and initiates an 80-joule charge. An 80-joule charge occurs within 10 seconds at beginning of life. After the capacitor charge is complete, *shock confirmation* (three fast intervals and sustained tachycardia) ensures the arrhythmia is sustained and appropriate to treat. An average time to therapy with the SICD is 15±3 seconds.

On this stored episode, the entire arrhythmia lasts 17.5 seconds. Sensing the arrhythmia and tachyarrhythmia detection occur in 9.5 seconds. The 80-joule charge is 8 seconds. Reconfirmation occurs, therapy is delivered, and the arrhythmia is converted. This is an appropriate time to therapy for the SICD.

During the detection phase, the SICD detects cardiac signals and adjusts sensitivity on a beat-to-beat basis. This allows appropriate sensing of sinus rhythm and increasing sensitivity to detect fine ventricular fibrillation. Additionally, the device uses filtering to prevent artifact or noise to be detected as a tachyarrhythmia. The SICD calculates the estimated peak of the R wave based on the average of the two previous peak values. The benefit is that a single event will not affect the detection profile. However, at the onset of an arrhythmia, a rapid decrease in the peak R-wave amplitude may require several R-R intervals in order for the estimated peak values to be averaged. R-wave undersensing (or dropout) may be seen early in the episode until peak averages are maximized with increased sensitivity, resulting in consistent sensing and tachyarrhythmia detection.

This phenomenon is noted at the beginning of this stored episode. Here, seven beats of the tachycardia occur before consistent R-wave sensing is marked. In addition, the SICD uses an average of four R-R intervals. The first "T" or tachycardia sensed marker is the fifth tachycardia event sensed by the SICD. Although initial arrhythmia dropout occurs briefly on the strip, this does not significantly delay detection.

While this patient's arrhythmia is detected in the shock zone, the SICD utilizes discriminators in the conditional (VT) zone. The device utilizes three criteria for VT versus SVT analysis. First, the device compares the waveform of the tachyarrhythmia event to a stored template. If >50% correlated, this suggests an SVT. If <50%, the SICD compares the current beat to the previous beat. If the two events are dissimilar, a polymorphic arrhythmia is suspected and therapy decision tree initiates. If the two events are similar, a VT is suspected and further analysis occurs. Last, the device compares the QRS width of the current tachyarrhythmia event to the stored template. If it is wide, VT is suspected; if narrow, an atrial arrhythmia is suspected.

Figure 4.A.2

Stored EGM, part 2.

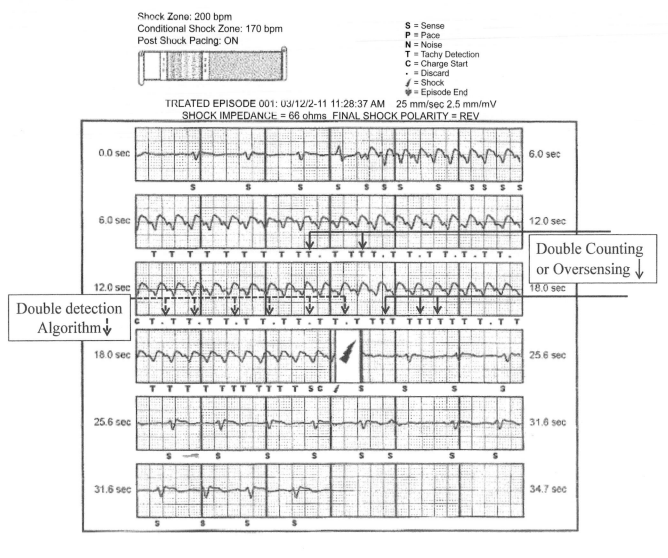

Figure 4.A.3

Cameron x-ray with annotations.

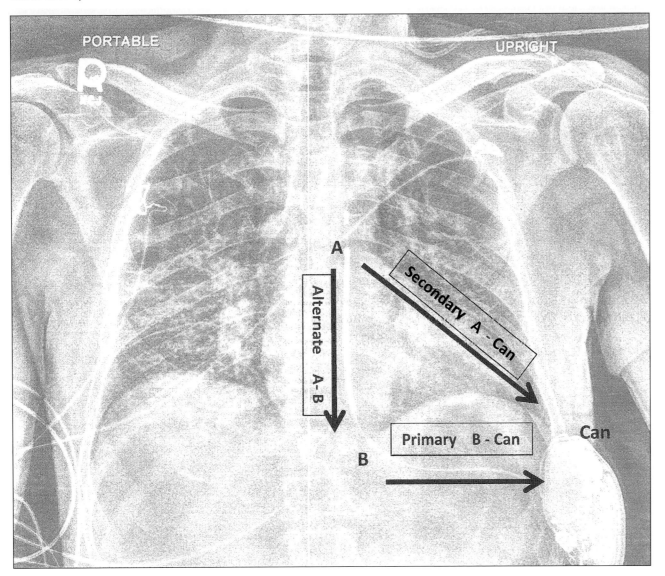

Figure 4.A.4

Conditional zone markers.

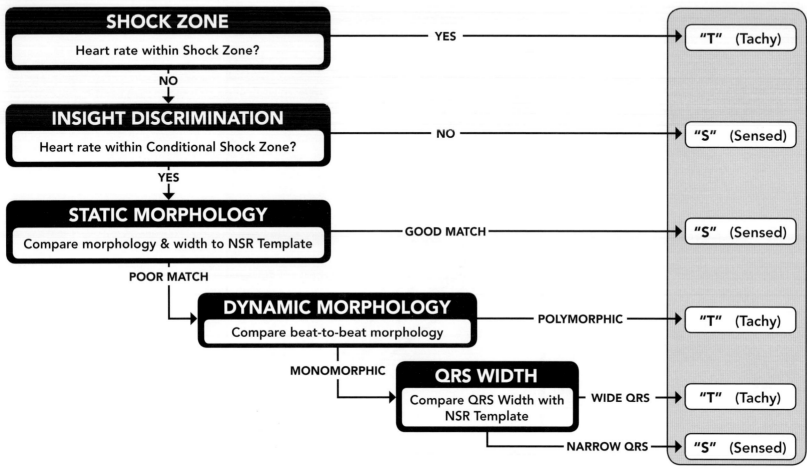

Figure 37: Decision Phase arrhythmia analysis

Source: Used with permission from Boston Scientific.

Reference

1. Gold MR, Theuns DA, Knight BP, et al. Head to head comparison of arrhythmia discrimination performance of subcutaneous and transvenous ICD arrhythmia detection algorithms: the START study. *J Cardiovasc Electrophysiol.* 2012;23(4):359-366.

2. Cameron Health Technical Memo—S-ICD System Algorithm Overview, DN-12345, Revision D:13-34.

Case 4.B

Background

A 52-year-old undergoes implantation of biventricular ICD. Pre-discharge interrogation shows pacing in the ventricle less than 50%. A rhythm strip from the device interrogation is shown.

Programmed Settings

DDD 60/120

SAV = 100 ms

PAV = 130 ms

PVARP = 310 ms

RA Lead: 3.5 V @ 0.4 ms, Sensitivity = 0.3 mV

RV Lead: 3.0 V @ 0.4 ms, Sensitivity = 0.3 mV

LV Lead: 6.0 V @ 1.1 ms

Question

What is causing the two sensed events following each paced event (BV)?

A) Two PVCs

B) PVC followed by intrinsic R wave

C) T-wave oversensing followed by intrinsic R wave

D) 60 Hz interference

Figure 4.B.1

EGM strip.

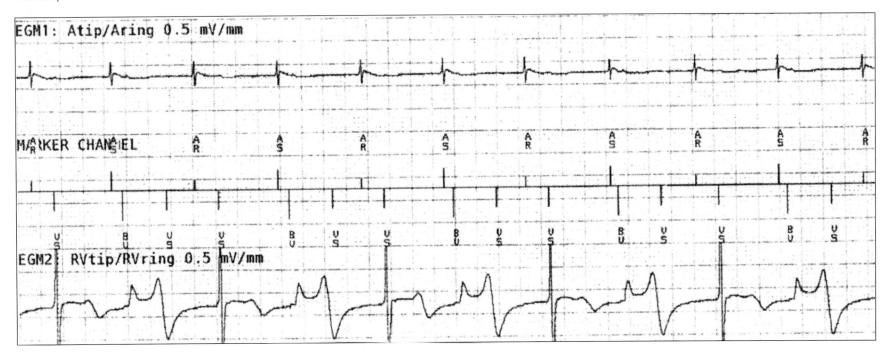

Answer

The correct answer is **C**. The two sensed events are the result of **T-wave oversensing followed by intrinsic R wave**.

The two VS markers following each paced event (BV) have very different morphologies. The first VS lines up with the T wave on the marker channel; the pattern is consistent for each beat (not a PVC). The second VS is very narrow and not likely a PVC. There is no evidence of 60-Hz EMI.

The T wave following the biventricular pace (BV) depolarization is sensed as the first VS. There is no atrial event between the BV and this first VS; therefore, the device defines this as a PVC and the Post-Ventricular Atrial Refractory Period (PVARP = 310 ms) is extended. The subsequent atrial event falls into refractory. The refractory event is not tracked and the next VS is an intrinsically activated R wave. The next P wave falls outside the PVARP, is tracked, and the pattern repeats itself.

Large T waves can be due to patient conditions (eg, hyperkalemia) or device conditions (eg, signal processing of signals). T-wave oversensing can often be corrected by reprogramming the device to a less sensitive setting. In order for this to be effective, the intrinsic signal must be sufficiently large.

Generally, reprogramming for T wave oversensing is different for devices with only pacing therapy versus those with defibrillating capability as follows:

1. Typically, pacemakers use a fixed sensitivity setting, while defibrillators use a dynamic sensitivity that decays with time to allow for fine sensing of VF.

2. Further precautions should be used if the device is an ICD, since adjusting the sensitivity can affect arrhythmia detection. If the device is made less sensitive, additional DFT testing should be considered. Recently, there have been algorithms developed that use frequency analysis to filter T waves independent of the sensitivity setting.

3. In this case, the overall percentage of CRT therapy is reduced due to oversensing. By reprogramming the sensitivity to 0.6 mV, we were able to successfully filter the T wave and restore consistent CRT therapy. DFT testing was performed at the new setting, and no undersensing of ventricular arrhythmias occurred.

Figure 4.B.2

Annotated EGM strip.

- The first VS following BV pace is due to oversensing of a T wave.
- Subsequent P wave falls in PVARP and is not tracked. Thus, intrinsic R wave is conducted (VS).
- The next P wave falls outside PVARP, is tracked, and the sequence repeats.

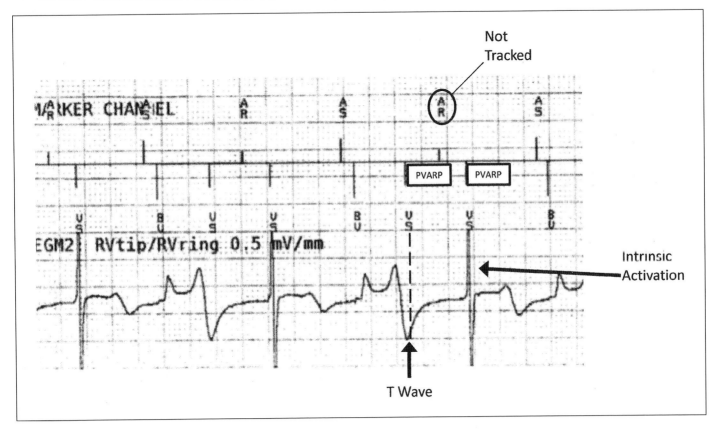

Figure 4.B.3

EGM strip with ventricular sensitivity reprogrammed to 0.45 mV.

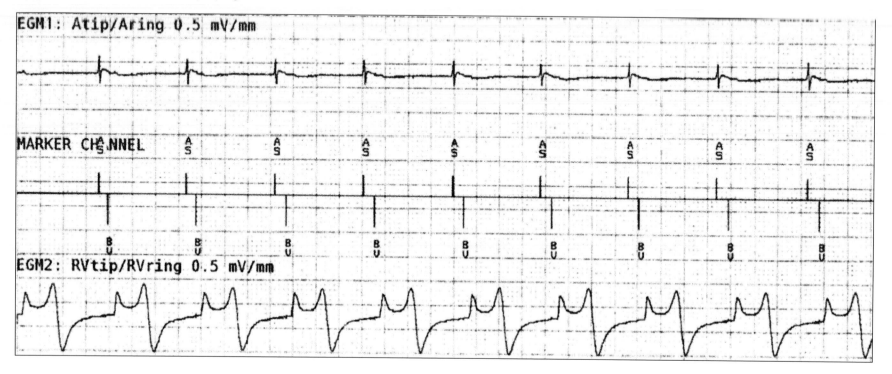

Reference

1. Seegers J, Vollman D, et al. Ventricular oversensing due to manufacturer-related differences in implantable cardioverter-defibrillator signal processing and sensing lead properties. *Europace*. 2010; 12(10):1460-1466.

2. Gold MR, et al. Head-to-head comparison of arrhythmia discrimination performance of subcutaneous and transvenous ICD arrhythmia detection algorithms: the START study. *J Cardiovasc Electrophysiol*. 2012;23:359-366.

Case 4.C

Background

A 62-year-old patient with a history of heart failure underwent implantation of a biventricular ICD two years ago. Due to unsatisfactory electrical performance, a new atrial lead is implanted. The next day, telemetry shows high rates with no pacing occurring.

Programmed Settings

DDD 70/120

SAV = 100 ms

PAV = 130 ms

PVARP = 310 ms

RA: 3.5V @ 0.4 ms, Sensitivity = 0.3 mV

RV: 2.5V @ 0.4 ms, Sensitivity = 0.3 mV

LV: 3V @ 0.6 ms

Table 4.C.1 ICD Detection Zone and Counter Settings

	Initial	Redetect	Interval
VF	18/24	9/12	300 ms
FVT			280 ms
VT	16	12	360 ms

Question

What is the most likely cause of the A-A interval pattern displayed in the interval plot above?

A) T-wave oversensing

B) Electromagnetic interference on the atrial channel

C) Far-field R-wave oversensing

D) Loose set screw on the atrial lead

Figure 4.C.1

Interval plot.

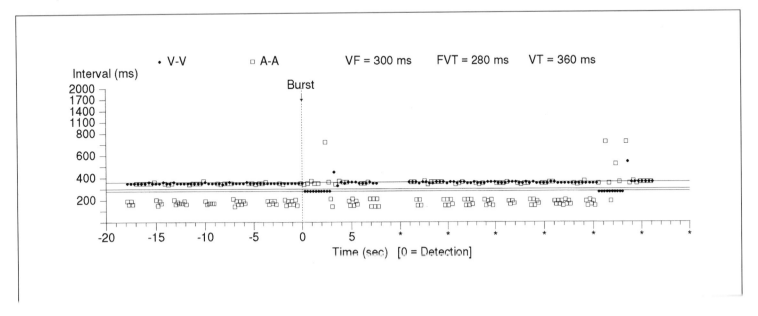

Answer

The correct answer is **C. Far-field R-wave oversensing** is responsible for the pattern shown.

On an interval plot, a "train track" pattern indicates repeating long-short intervals. The two common causes of this pattern are far-field R-wave (FFRW) oversensing and T-wave oversensing. FFRW oversensing shows a "train track" pattern of A-A intervals (squares on the interval plot), as R waves are oversensed on the atrial electrogram. T-wave oversensing would show a similar pattern in the V-V intervals (dots on the interval plot). Electromagnetic interference (EMI) shows a very fast and erratic pattern, which is not present in this case.

FFRW oversensing is unlikely to affect the pacing therapy of the device, as each oversensed R wave would fall into the programmed PVARP and be ignored. However, it does often affect tachycardia therapy. The high-power discriminators in ICDs use A-A and V-V interval patterns to distinguish VT/VF from an SVT. The patient was treated with burst ATP twice because the ventricular rate fell into the VT zone (≥167 bpm). We cannot know if this was a true VT or an SVT without further viewing the stored electrograms.

The FFRW oversensing pattern occurs in short runs roughly twice every 5 seconds on the interval plot. The frequency was confirmed to be due to the patient's respiratory rate as shown in the electrogram recording on the following page. The anode of atrial lead (placed in the atrial appendage) is moving during each breath. As it moves toward the ventricle, FFRW oversensing occurs.

FFRW oversensing can often be corrected by decreasing the sensitivity (ie, increasing the programmed sensitivity setting) of the atrial lead. This will only work provided that the sensed P waves have sufficiently larger amplitudes than the FFRWs. If the sensed P-wave amplitudes are small, the sensitivity should be increased (decreased programmed sensitivity setting) in order to have a consistent FFRW pattern. This will allow the ICD discriminators to better identify the pattern and withhold tachyarrhythmia therapy.

Reference

1. De Voogt WB, Van Hemel NM. Diagnostic tools for atrial tachyarrhythmias in implantable pacemakers: a review of technical options and pitfalls. *Neth Heart J.* 2008;16(6):201-210.

Figure 4.C.2

Annotated EGM strip.

- Each FFRW lines up with R waves on the ventricular electrogram.
- Oversensed FFRWs are labeled "AR" on the atrial electrogram because they fall into PVARP. Refractory events are ignored for pacing, but do count toward ICD discrimination.
- The additional "AR" makers create a repeating long-short (L-S-L-S) A-A interval pattern, which creates "train tracks" on the interval plot.
- Short runs of FFRW occur twice every five seconds due to respiratory movement of the atrial lead. The recording was made when the patient was instructed to take slow, deep breaths.

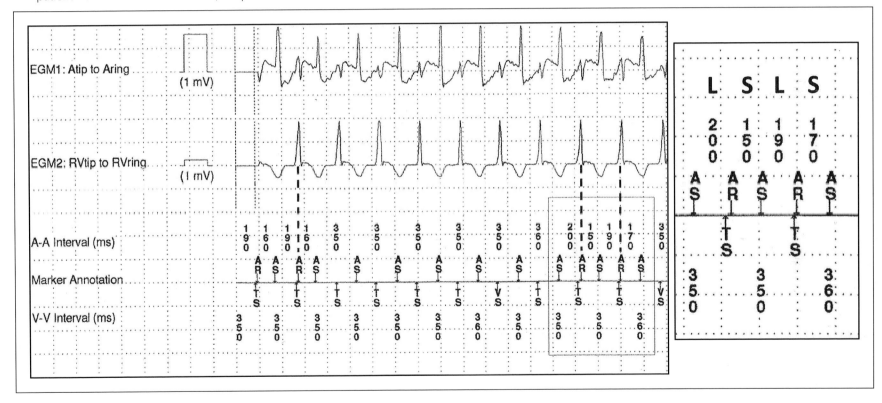

Case 4.D

Background

A 66-year-old male with previous MI and an EF of 25% was implanted with a Medtronic Maximo single-chamber ICD and a Sprint Fidelis 6949 (Medtronic Inc., Minneapolis, MN) high-voltage lead 2 years prior. The patient has no symptoms, but interrogation of the device indicates that there have been several nonsustained VT episodes.

Programmed Settings

VVI 40

RV: 2.5V @ 0.4 ms, Sensitivity = 0.3 mV

Table 4.D.1	ICD Detection Zone and Counter Settings		
	Initial	Redetect	Interval
VF	18/24	12/16	320 ms
FVT			280 ms
VT	16	12	360 ms

Question

What is the most likely explanation for the VF detection?

A) Noise on wavelet morphology discriminator

B) T-wave oversensing

C) Electromagnetic interference (EMI)

D) Both T-wave oversensing and noise on wavelet discriminator

Figure 4.D.1

EGM strip.

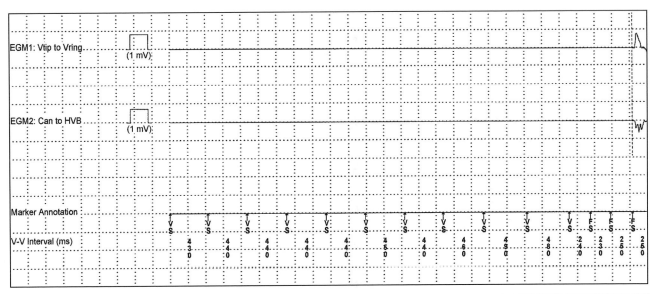

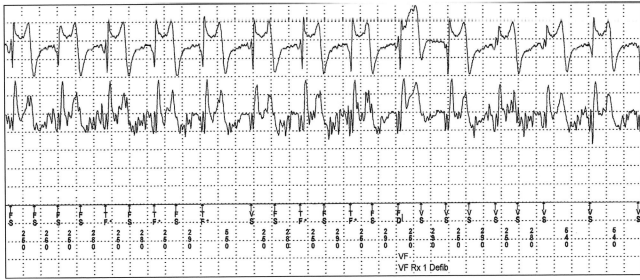

Figure 4.D.2

Interval plot.

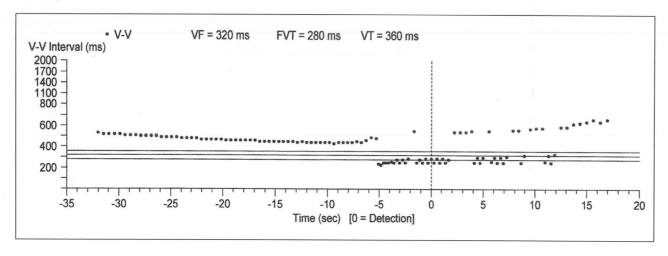

*A*nswer

The correct answer is **D. A combination of T-wave over-sensing and noise on wavelet discriminator** is responsible for VF detection.

The key is to understand the difference between the signals used by the device for detection and the signal source used by the discriminator. The device uses the Vtip–Vring circuit for sensing. Each sensed event is represented in the marker channel (at the bottom of Figure 4.D.1) and corresponds to the Vtip–Vring electrogram (EGM1), which shows no noise artifact. As shown in the annotation in Figure 4.D.4, each "FS" or or "FT" event

matches up with an R wave or T wave in EGM1, which is consistent with T-wave oversensing. This is also illustrated by the "train tracks" pattern on the interval plot. There is a consistent pattern of R-T interval then T-R interval that makes up each "rail" of the "train tracks." VF detection occurs when the VF counter reaches 18 (out of a window of 24).

The morphology discriminator, Wavelet, uses EGM2 (which is programmable) to discriminate SVTs from ventricular arrhythmias. In this case, EGM2 is a far-field source, Can-HVB (Can = device, HVB = distal coil, HVA = proximal coil), which displays noise artifact. Once the rhythm has reached detection (FD), Wavelet looks back at the previous 8 intervals, comparing the morphology of each R wave to a previously captured R-wave template (see see Figure 4.D.6).[1] A programmed match percentage allows for slight variations in morphology, while rejecting R waves that are distinctly different. The device will withhold therapy if at least 3 of the 8 intervals meet the match threshold. Because there is noise on the source electrogram, none of the 8 intervals matches the template, and VF detection is incorrectly confirmed.

Once detection occurred, the T-wave oversensing stopped, and the device aborted therapy. A fracture in the HVB conductor was suspected and supported by the spike in the HVB impedance.

Because the high-power circuit has been compromised, the patient was brought in for lead replacement.

If the integrity of lead had been acceptable, T-wave oversensing may have been filtered out by adjusting the ventricular sensitivity. Special precautions should be taken, as adjusting the sensitivity can affect the ability to detect arrhythmias; defibrillation testing should be repeated.

Reference

1. Klein GJ, Gillberg JM, et al. Improving SVT discrimination in single-chamber ICDs: A new electrogram morphology-based algorithm. *J Cardiovasc Electrophysiol.* 2006;17(12):1310-1319.

Figure 4.D.3

Train tracks on interval plot. The pattern of R-T interval then T-R interval creates two distinct and consistent "rails" of the "train tracks" displayed in the interval plot.

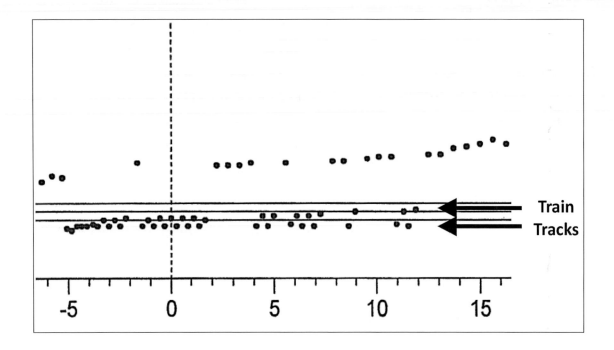

Figure 4.D.4

Each "FS" interval corresponds to an R wave, then a T wave. Note that the VTip-VRing electrogram is clean, while the Can-I IVB electrogram displays noise artifact.

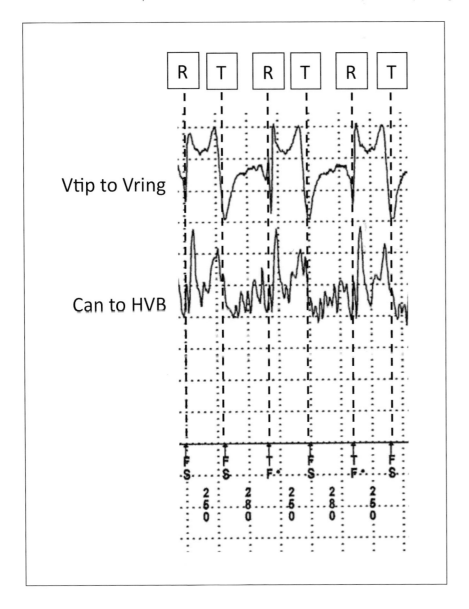

Figure 4.D.5

Can to HVB electrogram. Wavelet uses EGM2, which is nominally Can to HVB. At detection, the device compares the morphologies of the previous 8 intervals to a stored template. If ≥3 of 8 exceed match threshold (nominally 70%), therapy is withheld.

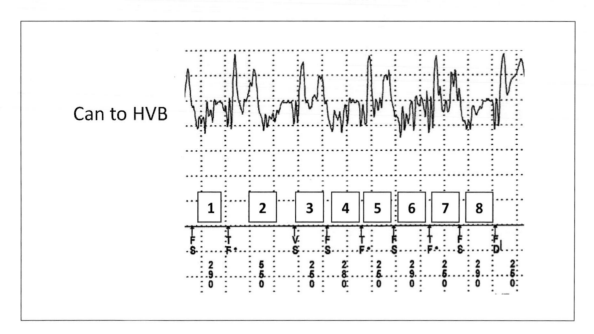

Figure 4.D.6

Wavelet match results. None of the 8 intervals matched due to noise artifact.

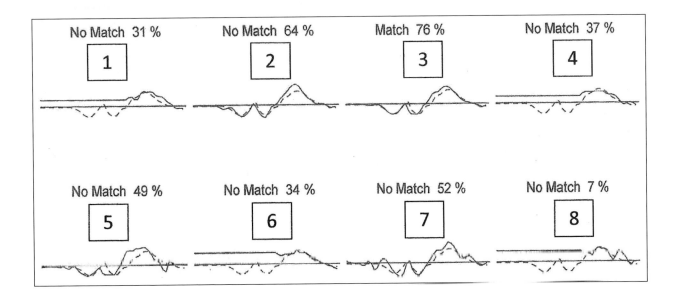

Background

A 44-year-old male with a history of sick sinus syndrome is implanted with a Medtronic Adapta (Medtronic Inc., Minneapolis, MN) dual-chamber pacemaker. The patient is held overnight for observation. Figure 4.E.1 shows a recorded telemetry strip.

Programmed Settings

AAIR↔DDDR (MVP Mode) 70/120

PAV = 280 ms

SAV = 250 ms

RA Lead: 2.5 V @ 0.4 ms, Sensitivity = 0.5 mV

RV Lead: 2.5 V @ 0.4 ms, Sensitivity = 4.0 mV

Question

Which of the following is the most likely explanation for each of the two 80-ms backup pacing spikes (denoted by asterisk)?

A) Ventricular undersensing, then atrial loss of capture

B) Functional ventricular undersensing, then atrial loss of capture

C) Ventricular safety pacing for both events

Figure 4.E.1

Telemetry strip.

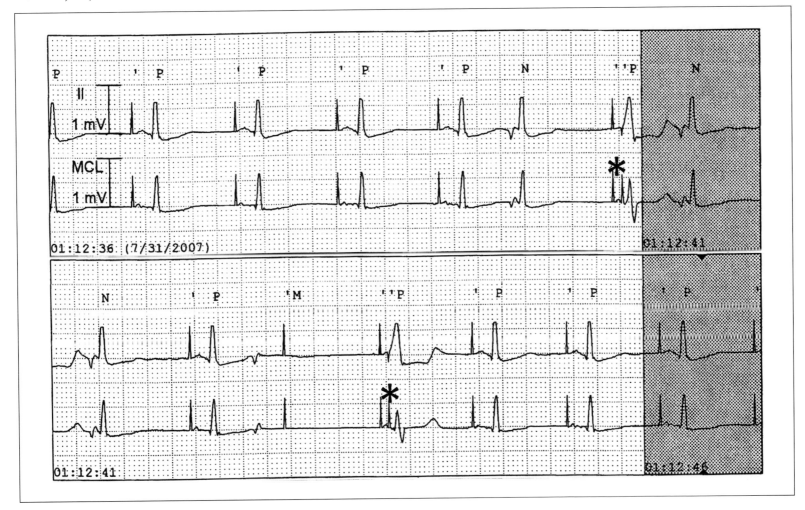

Answer

The correct answer is **B. Functional undersensing, then atrial loss of capture**, is the most likely explanation for these backup pacing spikes.

The 80-ms backup pacing distinguishes Managed Ventricular Pacing (MVP) operation from ventricular safety pacing (which is typically 100–110 ms). MVP will deliver ventricular backup pacing on the interval following a ventricular dropped beat. The dropped beat is defined as two consecutive atrial events with no ventricular event in between. Two of four intervals with ventricular dropped beats will result in a mode switch to DDD.

The first backup pace is due to functional undersensing of the preceding ventricular event: a PVC. The PVC occurs directly after a P wave and falls into the atrial blanking period (ABP). We know the P wave was sensed appropriately because the interval from the P wave to the next atrial pacing spike matches the lower rate interval (LRI) of 857 ms. The ventricular channel (on Adapta) has variable 50- to 70-ms ABP during sensed atrial events (MVP only). The PVC falls within the ABP and is not sensed. The device defines this as a dropped beat, and a ventricular backup paced beat is initiated on the next interval (see Figure 4.E.2).

The second backup pacing spike is due to atrial loss of capture. There is a PAC in the preceding interval that falls into atrial refractory period. In this case, auto-PVARP encompasses ~75% of the A–A timing cycle. The refractory PAC is not tracked, and the ensuing atrial pace is unable to capture because the tissue is now refractory. Neither the PAC nor the atrial pace is conducted to the ventricle, resulting in a dropped beat.

The timing cycles are illustrated in the Figure 4.E.3.

Figure 4.E.2

First backup ventricular pace.

- PVC being blanked and functionally undersensed; the device labels this as a dropped beat.
- After the PVC, the LRI times out, causing an atrial pace and ventricular backup pace with an 80-ms AV delay.

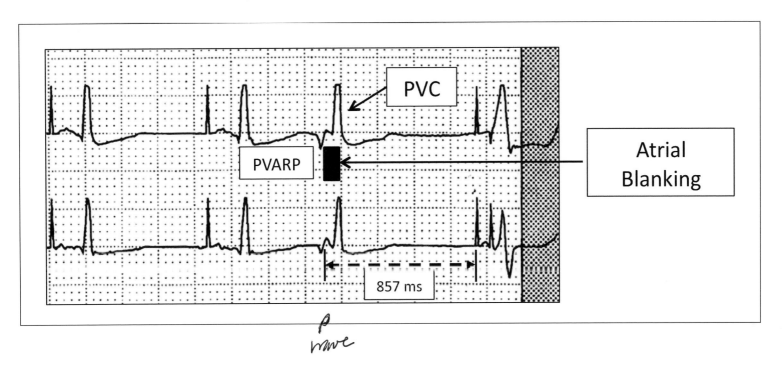

Figure 4.E.3

Second backup ventricular pace.

- A PAC falls into PVARP and is ignored.
- The LRI times out, resulting in an A pace with no conduction (tissue refractory) due to functional noncapture.
- The following interval is an A pace with ventricular backup pace.

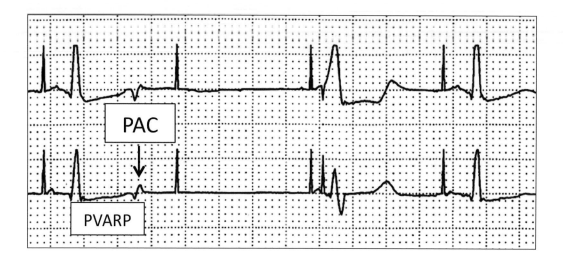

Reference

1. Sweeney MO, Sheldon T, et al. Randomized pilot study of a new atrial-based minimal ventricular pacing mode in dual-chamber implantable cardioverter-defibrillators. *Heart Rhythm*. 2004;1:160–167.

Case **4.F**

Background

A 56-year-old female with a history of syncope, negative tilt-table test, and a negative Holter monitor is implanted with a Reveal DX (Medtronic, Inc. Minneapolis, MN) implantable loop recorder (ILR). She visits the clinic for a device interrogation after several syncopal episodes. There are several recorded episodes. The following is an episode "marked" symptomatic by the patient with their associated handheld indicator.

Table 4.F.1	Programmed Settings	
	Initial	**V Interval**
FVT	12/16	300 ms
VT	16	360 ms
Asystole	3 sec	
Brady	4 beats	2000

Question

Which of the following is the most likely explanation for the abnormalities recorded by this tracing?

A) Asystole

B) Undersensed VF

C) Undersensed normal sinus rhythm

D) Electrostatic noise

Figure 4.F.1

EGM strip.

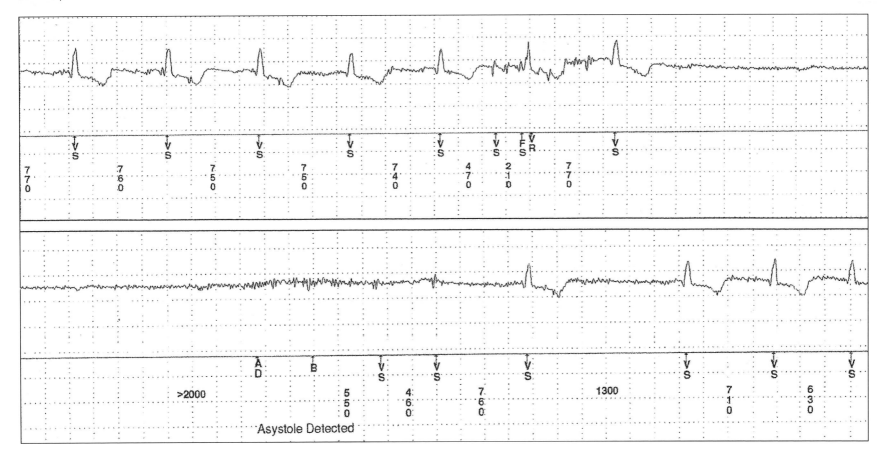

*A*nswer

The correct answer is **A. Asystole** is the most likely explanation

There is consistent noise and oversensing throughout both rhythm strips. On the first strip, each R wave is accounted for, and there are two instances of oversensing (see asterisks in Figure 4.F.2). After the seventh beat, there is an asystolic event greater than 4 seconds, which is broken up by oversensing of noise marked "B" for brady interval. There are two more oversensed events (marked as "VS") followed by a true R wave. In actuality, there is an approximately 6-second pause between R waves.

The signal-to-noise ratio remains high throughout both strips. The noise during asystole appears consistent with the noise during the normal sinus rhythm portions; this is not VF. In addition, there is no evidence of undersensing of R waves. If there were inconsistent electrode contact with tissue, you would see varying R-wave amplitudes, which is not present in this case.

Undersensing can be problematic in Reveal devices due to inconsistent contact of electrodes with subcutaneous tissue. As the device moves and the electrodes begin to separate from tissue, the strength of the signal decreases. The decreasing signal amplitude can result in undersensing. Subcutaneous implantation of the device in a tight pocket is necessary to prevent migration and separation of electrodes from tissue. Newer generations of loop recorders use auto-adjusting sensitivity algorithms similar to those in ICDs to better account for dynamic signal amplitudes. These dynamic sensing thresholds help prevent T-wave oversensing, yet still decay to allow for changes in R-wave amplitude.[1]

As a result of the Reveal recording, the patient was implanted with a dual-chamber pacemaker. The device was programmed with a rate-drop algorithm that paces only when syncope is present and for a programmable amount of time.

Reference

1. Brignole M, et al. Improved arrhythmia detection in implantable loop recorders. *J Cardiovasc Electrophysiol*. 2008;19(9):928-934.

Figure 4.F.2

Annotated EGM strip. Noise is present during normal sinus rhythm and during asystole. This is not VF, and there is no evidence of undersensing. Oversensed events are asterisked.

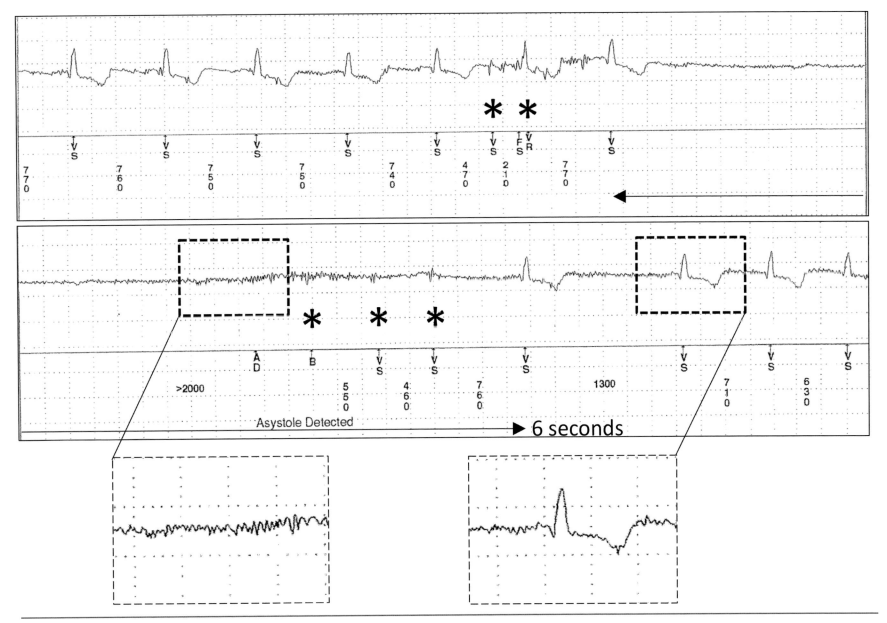

Case **4.G**

Background

A 71-year-old male with a history of sick sinus syndrome has a Medtronic EnPulse pacemaker (Medtronic Inc., Minneapolis, MN). The patient is hospitalized for a noncardiac procedure, but is monitored on telemetry. The following strip in Figure 4.G.1 is recorded.

Programmed Settings

DDDR 70/120

PAV = 200 ms

SAV = 170 ms

RA Lead: 2.5 V @ 0.4 ms, Sensitivity = 0.35 mV

RV Lead: 2.5 V @ 0.4 ms, Sensitivity = 2.8 mV

Question

What is the most likely cause of this rhythm?

A) Managed ventricular pacing

B) Atrial undersensing causes ventricular safety pacing

C) Ventricular undersensing causes ventricular safety pacing

Figure 4.G.1

Telemetry strip.

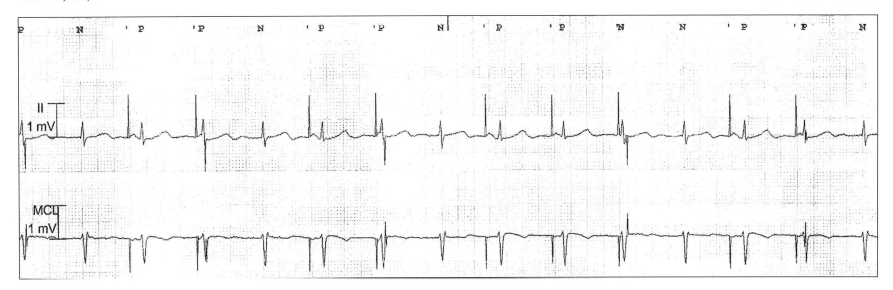

Answer

The correct answer is **B. Atrial undersensing** has caused the device to initiate ventricular safety pacing.

Ventricular safety pacing (VSP) typically has a 100- to 110-ms AV delay (Medtronic pacemakers use 110 ms), which is displayed in this strip. Managed ventricular pacing uses a backup ventricular pace 80 ms after a scheduled atrial pace only after a ventricular dropped beat. Neither of these criteria is met in the current case.

The lower rate interval (LRI, defined by the sensor-indicated, A-A pacing interval = 800 ms or 75 bpm) and the intrinsic rate (R-R interval = 700 ms or 85 bpm) are consistent throughout, which suggests that the patient is in normal sinus rhythm and that atrial pacing is occurring at a rate slower than his intrinsic rhythm. There is evidence of appropriate ventricular sensing on all beats, including VSP events (mistaking the R wave for crosstalk causes VSP). Thus, the most likely cause of the VSP is atrial undersensing. This can be proven by mapping out the timing intervals as shown in Figure 4.G.2.

There is a regular pattern that begins with atrial capture followed by an intrinsic R wave. On the next beat, atrial undersensing occurs (P wave is too small to see on the monitor strip) and the scheduled atrial pace occurs right before the conducted, intrinsic R wave. Because the R wave falls within 110 ms of the atrial pace, a safety pace occurs directly after the R wave. The LRI is preserved following the VSP, so the V-A interval is lengthened to 690 ms (LRI − 110 ms). Next, another undersensed P wave occurs, followed by an intrinsic R wave, which falls just prior to the V-A interval timing out. The device defines this as a PVC (ventricular event with no corresponding atrial event) and switches to modified atrial-based timing for this one beat. This will preserve the following V-A interval (LRI − PAV = 600 ms). After this 600-ms V-A interval, an atrial capture occurs, and the pattern will eventually repeat itself.

VSP is designed to prevent inappropriate inhibition of ventricular pacing due to crosstalk. Crosstalk occurs when the ventricular channel inappropriately senses the atrial pacing stimulus. Crosstalk in patients with no underlying ventricular rhythm could result in asystole. In this case, the R wave is mistaken as crosstalk, and the VSP falls harmlessly in the ventricular refractory period.

Further lead testing during interrogation revealed intermittent atrial sensing (P waves 0.3–0.4 mV) with appropriate atrial capture (threshold = 1.5 V at 0.4 ms). Appropriate atrial sensing was restored by increasing the atrial sensitivity; the sensitivity setting was reprogrammed from 0.35 mV to 0.25 mV.

Reference

1. Ellenbogen KA, Kay GN, Lau C, Wilkoff BL, eds. *Clinical Cardiac Pacing and Defibrillation*, 2nd ed. Philadelphia: Saunders Elsevier, 2007: 735-741.

Figure 4.G.2

Annotated telemetry strip.

1. The lower rate interval (800 ms) begins with atrial capture and an intrinsic R wave.

   - The intrinsic rate is 85 bpm (R-R interval, 700 ms).

2. The following P wave (not visible) is undersensed, causing the atrial pacing spike to fall right before the intrinsic R wave. The R wave falls into VSP window, and VSP occurs at 110 ms following atrial pace to prevent possible crosstalk inhibition.

   - The V-A interval following VSP is 690 ms (LRI – 110 ms).

3. The following P wave is undersensed, and the intrinsic R wave times out before scheduled atrial pace.

   - This is defined as a PVC, and modified atrial-based timing occurs for one beat, preserving the V-A interval = LRI – PAV (800 – 200 = 600 ms).

   - After this V-A interval times out, atrial capture occurs, and the pattern is repeated.

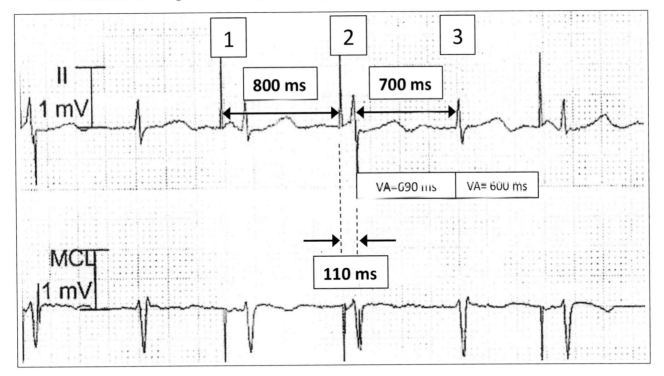

Case 4.H

Background

A 68-year-old male was evaluated in the emergency room for near-syncope. Patient history included a biventricular ICD generator implanted one month previously for ischemic cardiomyopathy, ejection fraction of 25%, NYHA Class III CHF, and complete heart block.

Programmed Settings

DDD 60–130 bpm

RA	2.0 V @ 0.5 ms	AGC 0.25 mV (Nominal)
RV	3.0 V @ 0.5 ms	AGC 0.6 mV (Nominal)
LV	3.0 V @ 0.5 ms	AGC 1.0 mV (Nominal)

Table 4.H.2 Lead Measurements

	Sensing	Impedance	HV	Threshold
RA	5.6	573 Ω		0.6 V @ 0.5 ms
RV	Paced	482 Ω	53 Ω	0.9 V @ 0.5 ms
LV	Paced	602 Ω		1.2 V @ 0.5 ms

Interrogation of the device reveals the stored NSVT electrogram in Figure 4.H.1.

Table 4.H.1 Tachycardia Parameters

	Duration	ATP	Shocks
VF >220 bpm	1.0 second	ATP × 1	21 J × 1; 41 J × 7
VT >170 bpm	2.5 seconds	ATP × 3 Scan	21 J × 1; 41 J × 5

Figure 4.H.1

Stored NSVT electrogram.

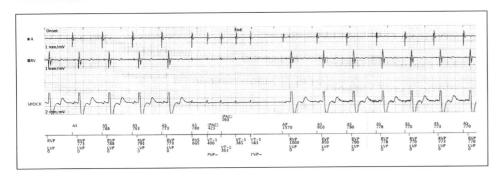

Question

What is the cause of this stored episode?

A) Nonsustained VT

B) Crosstalk

C) Far-field P-wave oversensing

D) Ventricular set screw issue

E) Ventricular lead fracture

Answer

The correct answer is **C**. The cause is **far-field P-wave oversensing** on the ventricular channel.

Figure 4.H.1 shows the following:

1. Short run of SVT, with minimal variation in the atrial electrogram (EGM) morphology.

2. Change in pattern on RV EGM; we no longer see large artifact on RV channel.

3. Small artifact noted on shock EGM, but it is inconsistent with ventricular depolarization and the timing matches up with RV EGM and RA EGM.

4. AS and VS markers occur concurrently.

With an integrated bipolar ICD lead, the sensing circuit consists of the tip electrode and the distal coil. If the RV ICD distal coil is positioned close to the tricuspid valve or if a micro-dislodgement occurs, the device may sense atrial signals/events on the ventricular channel. This may result in VT or VF detection and inappropriate therapy delivery. In a pacemaker-dependent patient, far-field P-wave oversensing may result in pacing inhibition and potential for syncope.

The stored EGM is not nonsustained VT. While there is a small artifact on the RV EGM, the shock EGM shows no ventricular depolarization. In fact, the morphology of the depolarization on the shock EGM demonstrates ventricular oversensing of an atrial signal.

Crosstalk is ventricular oversensing an atrial pacing electrical stimulus and pacing inhibition. In this case, the oversensing corresponds with an atrial sensed event on the ventricular channel, and thus cannot represent crosstalk.

With a new implant, a loose set screw may manifest as oversensing, exhibited by high-frequency, rapid, nonphysiologic signals. Generally, a loose set screw presents with a very high pacing impedance. Here, the pacing impedance and threshold were within normal limits and therefore do not likely reflect a set screw issue. Additionally, the signal seen on the RV EGM is most consistent with atrial activity, based on timing and amplitude reduction. The possibility of a patient simultaneously experiencing an exact increase in the atrial and ventricular cycle length is unlikely.

An RV lead fracture would be unlikely one month post-device implant; moreover, lead measurements are not consistent with a fracture.

Figure 4.H.2

Enlarged stored EGM. Note the small artifacts noted on the RV EGM and shock EGM channels consistent with sensed atrial activity by the ICD (ventricular) lead.

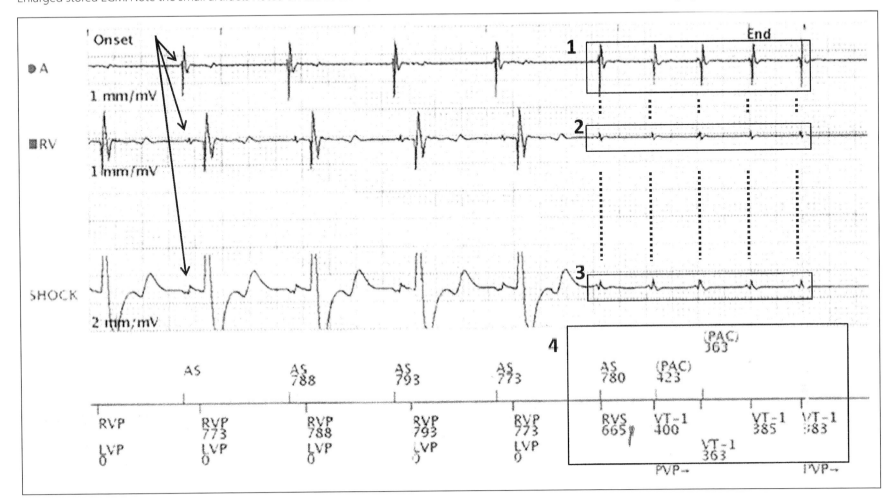

Figure 4.H.3

True bipolar ICD lead.

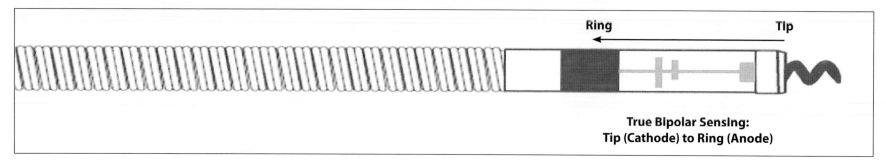

True Bipolar Sensing:
Tip (Cathode) to Ring (Anode)

Figure 4.H.4

Integrated bipolar ICD lead.

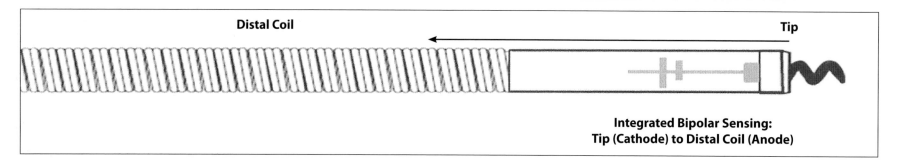

Integrated Bipolar Sensing:
Tip (Cathode) to Distal Coil (Anode)

Although far-field P-wave oversensing is more likely to occur with an integrated bipolar lead due to a larger sensing antenna, it may still occur with a dedicated bipolar lead. This is more likely to occur with a lead dislodgement. Programming the device to a lower sensitivity may effectively minimize P-wave oversensing. In some devices, a manual measurement of the far-field signal may be obtained from the ICD to assist in programming to avoid oversensing. DFT testing should be performed at the less sensitive setting to evaluate ICD sensing and appropriate VF detection. Far-field P-wave oversensing requiring ICD lead repositioning is rare.

References

1. Swerdlow CD, Gillberg JM, Khairy P. Sensing and detection. In: Ellenbogen KA, Kay GN, Lau CP, Wilkoff BL, eds. *Clinical Cardiac Pacing, Defibrillation, and Resynchronization Therapy*, 4th edition. Philadelphia: Elsevier Saunders, 2011:56-126.

2. Weretka S, Michaelsen J, Becker R, et al. Ventricular oversensing: a study of 101 patients implanted with dual chamber defibrillators and two different lead systems. *Pacing Clin Electrophysiol.* 2003;26:65-70.

Case 4.1

Background

A 73-year-old female is admitted to the coronary care unit complaining of chest pain and shortness of breath. Her ejection fraction is 30%, decreased from 45% last year. a DDD pacemaker was implanted 4 years ago for symptomatic sick sinus syndrome.

The following information was noted from device interrogation.

Programmed Settings

DDD 60–110 bpm

AV delay Min 260 ms, Max 400 ms

PVARP Min 260 ms, Max 300 ms

Table 4.1.1 Programmed Parameters

	Amplitude	Pulse Width	Sensitivity
RA	2.0 V	0.1 ms	0.75 mV
RV	2.0 V	0.4 ms	2.0 ms

Table 4.1.2 Lead Measurements

	Sensing	Impedance	Threshold	% Paced
RA	2.8 mV	450 Ω	0.4 V @ 0.5 ms	73%
RV	8.4 mV	650 Ω	0.8 V @ 0.5 ms	26%

The following telemetry strip is noted while the patient is admitted in CCU (Figure 4.1.1).

Figure 4.1.1

Telemetry strip.

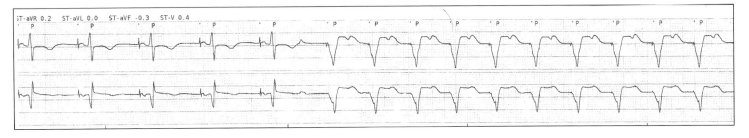

Question

What initiates this pacemaker mediated tachycardia?

A) Appropriate atrial sensing

B) Atrial undersensing

C) Atrial oversensing

D) Ventricular oversensing

Answer

The correct answer is **A. Appropriate atrial sensing** has taken place.

At the beginning of this strip, the device is atrial pacing with intact conduction. A PAC occurs that doesn't conduct. The AV delay times out to the maximum AV delay of 400 ms (the device is pacing at the LRL) and VP occurs. Because the AV delay is so long, the atria are no longer refractory, and a retrograde P wave occurs at a retrograde conduction time of 360 ms (see annotated Figure 4.I.2).

With the slow retrograde conduction time and the long AV delay, a PMT is induced at 90 bpm, well below the MTR. Because the device is not pacing at the MTR, the event is not categorized as PMT and the PMT algorithm is not initiated. The PMT algorithm is initiated with 16 AS/VP intervals at the MTR. On the next interval, the device extends the PVARP to 400 ms in an effort to terminate the tachycardia.

This patient's symptoms may be associated with loss of AV synchrony and long AV delays.

Reprogramming the device with a PVARP of 400 ms may effectively prevent PMTs. However, a longer PVARP and the current parameters (long AV delay) will significantly limit MTR. Given that this patient has intact conduction at 200 ms with RA pacing, a more appropriate option is to shorten the AV delay to 220 ms and PVARP to 400 ms.

Atrial undersensing does not occur. If the P wave had been undersensed, an atrial paced event would have occurred.

Atrial oversensing does not occur. If the P wave had been oversensed, the programmed AV delay would not have timed out.

Reference

1. Dennis M, Sparks P. Pacemaker mediated tachycardia as a complication of auto intrinsic conduction function. *Pacing Clin Electrophysiol.* 2004;27:824–826.

Figure 4.I.2

Annotated telemetry strip. (1) PAC occurs. (2) 400-ms AV delay times out and RV pace occurs. (3) Retrograde P wave occurs @ 360 ms outside Max PVARP 300 ms. (4) Device initiates PMT at 680 ms below maximal tracking rate (MTR) with AV delay 340 ms due to programmed dynamic AV.

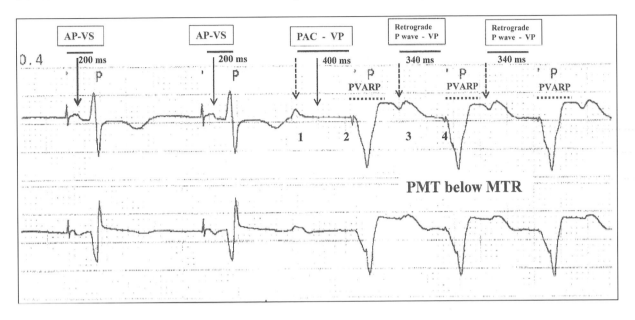

Case 4.J

Background

A 59-year-old female comes to the ER complaining of three episodes of near-syncope in the past week. She received a primary prevention ICD with a single coil lead 3 months ago for non-ischemic cardiomyopathy, ejection fraction of 25% and chronic atrial fibrillation. She is currently taking 200 mg metoprolol daily. ICD interrogation reveals 3 VF episodes, one of which resulted in defibrillation, and 7 NSVT episodes for which therapy was aborted. The stored EGMs are initiated with a similar pattern and are consistent with the time of the patient's symptoms. An example of this is seen in Figure 4.J.1.

Programmed Settings

VVI 40 bpm

3.5 V @ 0.5 ms

Sensitivity 0.6 mV AGC (Nominal)

Table 4.J.1 Tachycardia Parameters

VF	>220 bpm	DUR 7 seconds	31 J x x 1	41 J x 7
VT	>170 bpm	Monitor only		

Table 4.J.2 Lead Measurements

	Sensing	Impedance	HV	Threshold
RV	17 mV	533 Ω	77 Ω	0.7 V @ 0.5 ms

Figure 4.J.1

Onset.

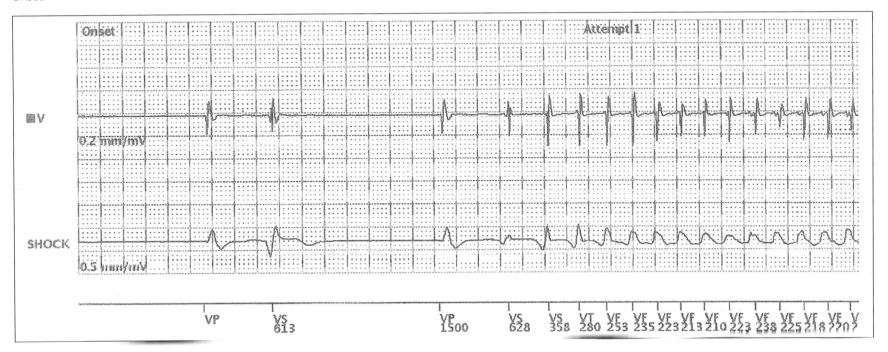

Question

What is the most appropriate course of action for this patient?

A) Catheter ablation of her ventricular tachycardia

B) Program bradycardia pacing "off" and decrease beta blocker dose

C) Initiate therapy with amiodarone

D) Reposition the ICD lead

Answer

The correct answer is **B**. The most appropriate course of action would be to **reprogram the device's bradycardia pacing mode to "off" and decrease the beta blocker dose**.

Ventricular arrhythmias may be induced by bradycardia or may be pause induced. In this scenario, the ventricular pace facilitates the ventricular arrhythmia by establishing a short–long–short sequence. The ventricular paced event actively initiates the ventricular arrhythmia. Reprogramming the device to minimize RV pacing negates the potential for further episodes. In this particular patient, it is hard to know how much of the problem is caused by right ventricular pacing and how much is due to the short–long–short sequence. By doing both—lowering the beta blockers and disabling pacing—the patient is likely to improve. If the patient needed pacing, an alternative solution would have been to program the pacing rate to 70 bpm or faster to avoid pauses. Reprogramming to OVO bradycardia mode will effectively decrease the risk of pacing-facilitated arrhythmias. It is necessary to know how programming the bradycardia pacing mode will affect postshock pacing. Are bradycardia pacing and postshock pacing consistent with programming changes? In addition, is postshock pacing necessary for this patient? Reviewing stored DFT testing data and episodes with defibrillation therapy provides additional information regarding the safety and efficacy of programming the bradycardia pacing to OVO.

At the next interrogation, patient symptoms and histogram data must be evaluated in terms of heart rate stability post-medication changes.

An ablation to treat this arrhythmia is not the best treatment for this patient. The rate of the tachycardia is 220 ms. Empiric amiodarone therapy will likely result in additional conduction issues and additional pacing for this patient. With the mechanism of ventricular pacing facilitating the arrhythmia, the likelihood of additional short–long–short sequences inducing VF may increase. Repositioning the ventricular lead will not resolve the problem of pacing-induced ventricular arrhythmia.

Reference

1. Sweeney MO, Ruetz LL, Belk P, Mullen TJ, Johnson JW, Sheldon T. Bradycardia pacing-induced short long short sequences at the onset of ventricular tachyarrhythmias: a possible mechanism of proarrhythmia. *J Am Coll Cardiol.* 2007;50:614–622.

Figure 4.J.2

Onset with annotations.

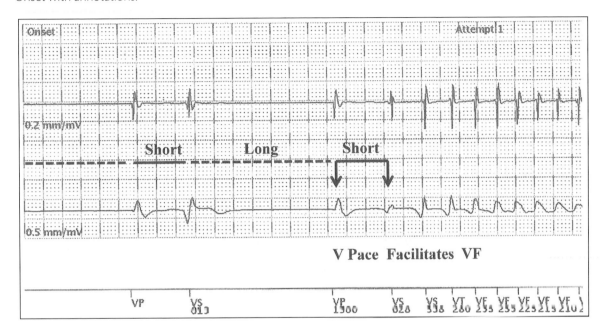

Case **4.K**

A 62-year-old female was admitted to the hospital for an ICD generator change. The ICD was implanted 5 years ago for an ischemic cardiomyopathy with an ejection fraction of 20% and ventricular tachycardia. DFTs at original implant were 14 joules. Daily pace/sense measurements have been consistent throughout the life of the device. Appropriate VT therapy has been delivered.

Programmed Settings

DDDR 60–120 bpm

RA	2.0 V @ 0.5 ms	AGC 0.18 mV (Nominal)
RV	4.0 V @ 0.5 ms	AGC 0.27 mV (Nominal)

Table 4.K.1 Tachycardia Parameters

VF	210 bpm	1 second duration		31 J × 8
VT	155 bpm	5 seconds duration	ATP × 6	14 J × 1, 31 × 5

Table 4.K.2 Lead Measurements

	Sensing	Impedance	HV	Threshold
RA	1.6 mV	345 Ω		0.6 V @ 0.5 ms
RV	5.6 mV	640 Ω	43 Ω	0.8 V @ 0.5 ms

During DFT testing, the ICD was programmed to least sensitive and a 14-J shock was programmed for the first therapy. A 1.1-J shock on T wave was used to induce VF. The resulting test strip is shown in Figure 4.K.1.

Figure 4.K.1

Least sensitive.

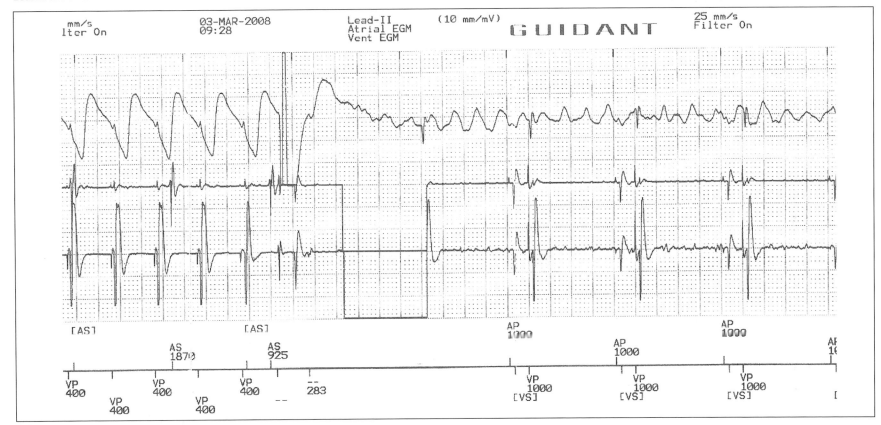

Question

The next appropriate step would be:

A) Retest DFT with a shortened ventricular blanking period

B) Retest DFT with a 50-Hz burst induction method

C) Retest DFT with a 310-ms coupling interval for the 1.1-J T shock

D) Retest at nominal sensitivity

Answer

The next appropriate step would be **D: retest DFT at nominal sensitivity**.

With the device programmed to least sensitive during DFTs, VF is not sensed, resulting in DDD pacing. A conservative approach to manage this patient, with chronic leads in place and consistent/stable lead measurements, would be to retest the DFT at a more sensitive setting to assess for appropriate VF detection and signal dropout. With appropriate detection and therapy, the final device programming can be programmed to "most" sensitive with a safety margin. When reprogrammed to nominal sensitivity and DFTs were retested, the device appropriately sensed VF.

A less conservative approach would be to implant a new RV rate/sense or a new ICD lead and retest DFTs. A venogram should be obtained to assess patency of the vein and may direct the course of action with chronic leads.

In the scenario of a new lead and a new ICD implant, undersensing of VF during DFT testing suggests the need to reposition the ICD lead and additional DFT testing. This should most commonly be a concern if the R wave during sinus rhythm is less than 5 mV. Changing the ventricular blanking period should have minimal effect on sensing ventricular fibrillation. The ventricular blanking period is the portion of the timing cycle after atrial pacing when the ventricular sense amplifier is not "open" to sensing ventricular signals. Because the cycle length of VF is so rapid, changing the blanking period is not likely to alter sensing. Because the QT interval is 340 ms, shortening the coupling interval to 310 ms may decrease the likelihood of inducing VF. Once again, this has no effect on sensing and VF detection. Inducing VF with a 50-Hz burst will not have any effect on sensing and detection.

Reprogramming the device to nominal sensitivity resulted in appropriate detection of ventricular fibrillation during additional DFT testing.

Figure 4.K.2

Nominal sensitivity.

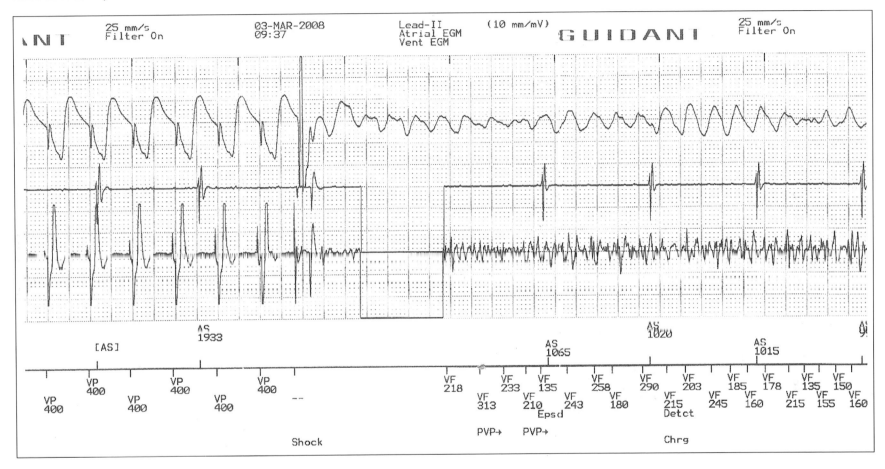

Figure 4.K.3

Least sensitive with annotations.

1. VF on surface ECG

2. RA EGM shows minimal low level-variation, but this is irrelevant because VF sensing and detection all based on the RV sensing.

3. RV EGM with low variation on baseline. This provides information regarding ventricular activity, but no intrinsic R-wave sensing occurs.

4. No P- or R-wave sensing occurs, resulting in AP and VP events and markers. [RV] markers annotate RV events in blanking, likely related to crosstalk with high output pacing postshock pacing.

Shock EGM may provide additional information regarding ventricular activity.

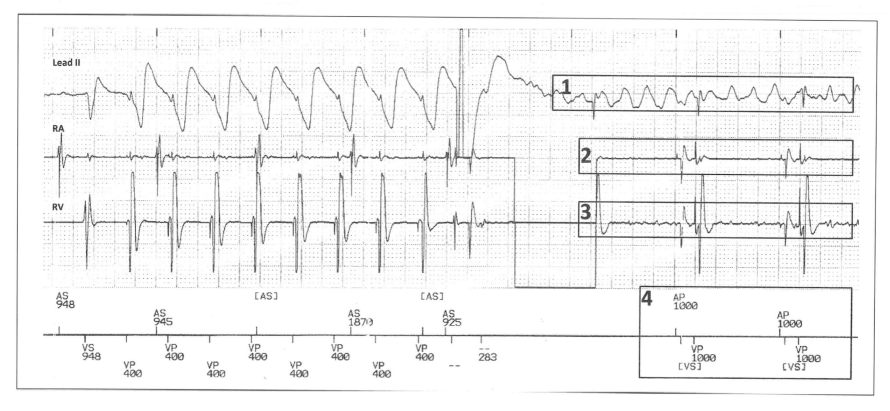

Reference

1. Swerdlow CD, Gillberg JM, Khairy P. Sensing and detection. In: Ellenbogen KA, Kay GN, Lau CP, Wilkoff BL, ed. *Clinical Cardiac Pacing, Defibrillation, and Resynchronization Therapy*, 4th edition. Philadelphia: Elsevier Saunders, 2011:56-126.

Case 4.L

Background

A 72-year-old male was evaluated in an ICD clinic during a follow-up visit. His ICD was implanted 4 years ago for an ischemic cardiomyopathy and an ejection fraction of 20%. His interrogation showed that he received ATP for ventricular tachycardia with successful termination of the arrhythmia. Multiple NSVT episodes are stored by device. The patient stated that he recently had a 4-day hospital admission for pneumonia.

Programmed Settings

DDD 50-120 bpm

RA 3.5 V @ 0.5 ms AGC 0.18 mV (Nominal) Sensitivity

RV 3.5 V @ 0.5 ms ACG 0.27 mV (Nominal) Sensitivity

Table 4.L.1 Tachycardia Parameters

VF 200 bpm	1 second DUR		21 J × 1, 41 J × 7
VT 175 bpm	2.5 second DUR	ATP × 3	5 J × 1, 21 J × 1, 41 J × 3
VT1 150 bpm	2.5 second DUR	ATP × 2	No shocks programmed

Table 4.L.2 Measured Data

	Sensing	Impedance	HV	Threshold
RA	2.6 mV	627 Ω		1.4 V @ 0.5 ms
RV	7.1 mV	411 Ω	HV 40 Ω	1.8 V @ 0.5 ms

The following stored episode (Figure 4.L.1) is typical of several NSVT episodes stored by the device.

Figure 4.L.1

Stored NSVT episode.

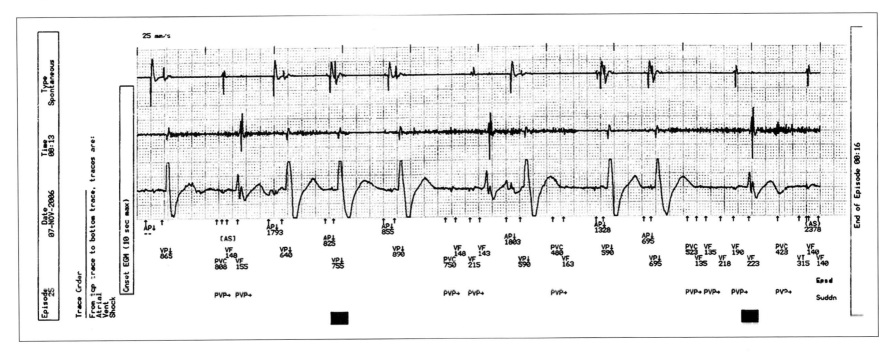

Question

What is the mechanism that caused the stored EGM?

A) RV lead fracture

B) Diaphragmatic oversensing

C) Pectoral muscle oversensing

D) Electromagnetic interference

E) High-voltage pins reversed in header

Answer

The correct answer is **B**. The mechanism for the stored episode is **diaphragmatic oversensing**.

Diaphragmatic oversensing is characterized by high-frequency and low-amplitude signals on the ventricular rate/sense EGM. This is generally seen with minimal variation in interval size, recognized as RV sensed events and may include VT/VF detection markers. This pattern is most commonly noted in patients with integrated bipolar ICD leads and apical lead placement. Additionally, respirophasic noise is often associated with ventricular pacing (VP) because the device is more likely to reach the maximum programmed sensitivity with an adjusting gain sensitivity device. The oversensing may result in VT or VF episode detection and an inappropriate shock and/or ventricular pacing inhibition. In pacemaker-dependent patients, they may present with near-syncope or syncope due to inhibition of pacing during the oversensing. Currently, this pattern of oversensing is rarely seen on Boston Scientific devices as a result of the nominal RV sensitivity programming at 0.6 mV and Dynamic Noise Algorithm.

The oversensing/noise is reproducible with deep breathing, coughing, or Valsalva maneuvers. Reprogramming the device to a less sensitive setting may effectively eliminate oversensing.

DFT testing should be performed with lower sensitivity to evaluate VF detection. If DFTs were previously tested at least sensitivity with appropriate sensing and detection, reprogramming can be done with confidence regarding arrhythmia detection. If oversensing persists with lower sensitivity settings, implanting a new pacing lead with RV septal placement is indicated.

At 4 years postimplant, RV lead fracture must be evaluated. The lead fracture is characterized by chaotic changes in the sensed ventricular electrogram with respect to timing and amplitude, and the variations can be striking. Additionally, there should be no "noise" on the far-field electrogram. In addition, lead measurements (eg, R wave and impedance) are consistently within normal limits.

Pectoral muscle myopotential oversensing is noted on the shock EGM only, not on the RV EGM. The low-level noise is found only on the shock EGM and is reproducible with isometrics. Since sensing only occurs from the RV EGM and not the shock EGM, there is no potential for inappropriate therapy.

Electromagnetic interference (EMI) oversensing is noted on all channels in a similar pattern. Depending on the source of EMI, the pattern may be high or low amplitude, but is repetitive in nature. RV oversensing may occur due to EMI with inappropriate VT/VF detection and inappropriate therapy.

When the high-voltage pins are reversed in the header, EGM characteristics on the shock EGM include prominent P waves and similar amplitude of the P and R wave. If high-voltage pins are reversed in a Guidant ICD, noise with varying amplitude may be reproducible with isometrics on the RV and shock EGM.

Figure 4.L.2

Diaphragmatic oversensing.

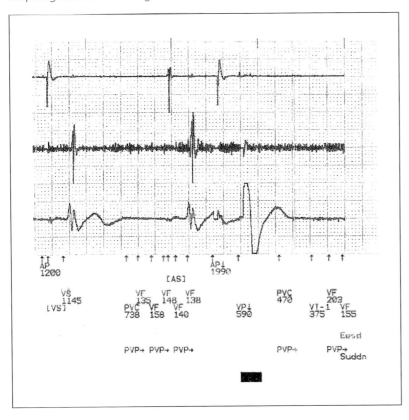

Figure 4.L.3

Pectoral muscle myopotential.

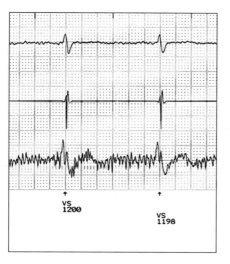

Figure 4.L.4

EMI.

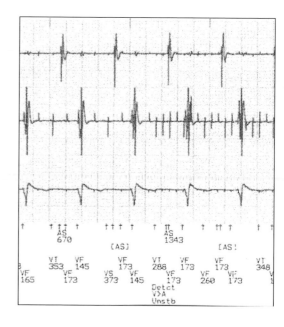

Figure 4.L.5

RV ICD rate sense fracture.

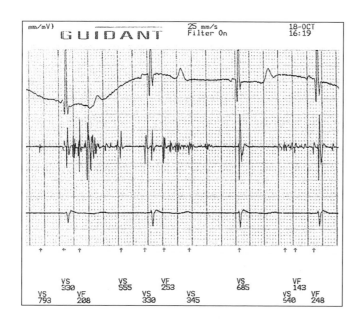

Figure 4.L.6

Proximal and distal coils reversed.

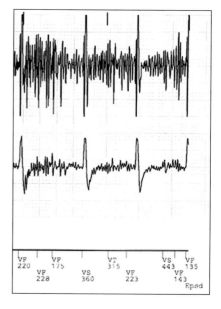

Reference

1. Sweeney MO, Ellison KE, Shea JB, Newell JB. Provoked and spontaneous high frequency, low amplitude, respirophasic noise transients in patients with implantable cardioverter defibrillators. *J Cardiovasc Electrophysiol.* 2001;12:402–411.

2. Kowalski M, Ellenbogen KA, Wood MA, Friedman P. Implantable cardiac defibrillator lead failure or myopotential oversensing? An approach to the diagnosis of noise on lead electrograms. *Europace.* 2008;10:914-917.

3. Pai RK, Abedin M, Rawling DA. Inappropriate ICD shocks for inappropriate reasons. *Indian Pacing Electrophysiol J.* 2008;8:69 71.

4. Weretka S, Michaelsen J, Becker R, et al. Ventricular oversensing: a study of 101 patients implanted with dual chamber defibrillators and two different lead systems. *Pacing Clin Electrophysiol.* 2003;26:65-70.

Case **4.M**

Background

A 59-year-old male was admitted to the emergency room c/o ICD discharge while mowing grass. A primary prevention ICD was implanted 6 weeks prior to ER admission for ischemic cardiomyopathy, ejection fraction of 25%, and NYHA Class II Heart Failure. Past medical history includes a CABG in 2007. The ICD interrogation shows 1 VF therapy, 6 VF episodes with diverted shocks, and 4 NSVT episodes over the past month. The patient has an integrated bipolar ICD lead. A stored VF episode, Figure 4.M.1, was recorded while the patient was mowing his lawn.

Programmed Settings

VVI 40 bpm

3.5 V @ 0.5 ms, AGC 0.27 mV (Nominal)

Table 4.M.1 Tachycardia Parameters

VF	210 bpm	1 seconds DUR		21 J × 1	31 J × 7
VT	190 bpm	6 seconds DUR	ATP × 3	11 J × 1	31 J × 5
VT1	170 bpm	8 seconds DUR	ATP × 6	11 J × 1	31 J × 5

Table 4.M.2 Measured Data

	Sensing	Impedance	High Voltage	Threshold
RV	4.9 mV	454 Ω	54 Ω	1.2 V @ 0.5 ms

Figure 4.M.1

Stored VF episode.

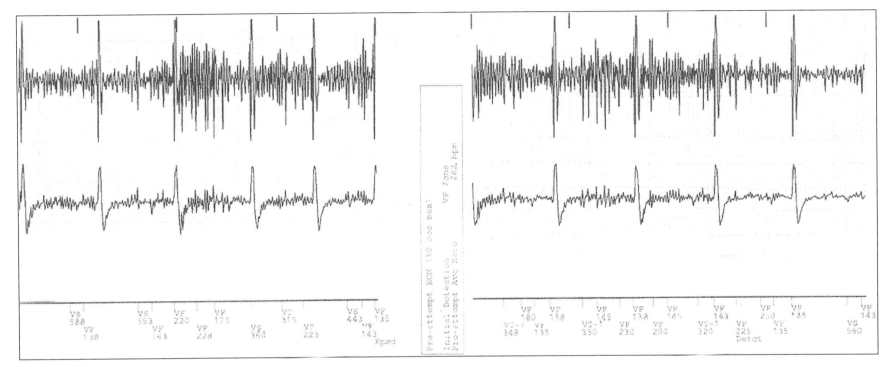

Question

What is the differential diagnosis for the stored episode?

A) High-voltage pins reversed in the header

B) Diaphragmatic oversensing

C) Pectoral myopotential oversensing

D) Loose set screw

E) ICD lead fracture

Answer

The answer is **A. High-voltage pins reversed in the header** is the appropriate differential diagnosis.

With an integrated bipolar lead, the sensing and pacing circuit is from the pacing tip to the distal shocking coil. If proximal and distal coils are reversed in the header of a Guidant ICD, an additional sensing configuration is now created with a larger antennae or sensing vector between the ICD tip and Can (because the Can and proximal coil were hardwired together). This unipolar sensing configuration may result in oversensing pectoralis muscle activity. As noted on the stored episode, inappropriate VF detection and therapy may result (Figure 4.M.2).

With high-voltage pins reversed in the header in older Guidant devices, it was common to see prominent P waves on the shock EGM and noise on the RV and shock EGM with varying amplitude, which are easily reproducible with isometrics. Regarding high-voltage therapy, when programmed to Initial HV Configuration, the energy is delivered from the distal coil to proximal coil and Can. If the proximal and distal pins are reversed, the high-voltage therapy will be delivered in a suboptimal vector. At implant, this often manifests with high DFTs. All lead measurements are within normal limits.

With Boston Scientific devices, the proximal coil and Can are not hardwired together. If the high-voltage pins are reversed, this eliminates the potential unipolar sensing configuration and avoids a risk of myopotential oversensing on the RV EGM.

In addition, the DF-4 ICD lead design eradicates the possibility of reversing the high-voltage pins.

Diaphragmatic oversensing is characterized with low-level noise on the RV EGM only. This noise pattern is reproduced with coughing or deep inspirations.

Pectoral muscle oversensing is noted on the shock EGM and may be reproduced with isometric activity. Because ICD sensing occurs on the rate sense portion of the system, oversensing does not occur, and inappropriate therapy will not be delivered in this scenario.

Given that the system has been implanted for only 6 weeks, failure of the set screw to be completely engaged must be considered. However, this can be ruled out by several pieces of data. Lead impedance measurements are within normal measurements. Additionally, a loose set screw would manifest as noise on the EGM to which it corresponds.

Similarly, it is unlikely to have a lead fracture as early as 6 weeks post initial implant. Lead measurements do not support a fracture. Unless the entire lead was fractured, there would not be noise on the RV and shock EGMs; the noise would manifest on the EGM that corresponds with the fractured conductor.

Figure 4.M.2

Physically reversing the DF-1 lead terminals with
an integrated bipolar lead.

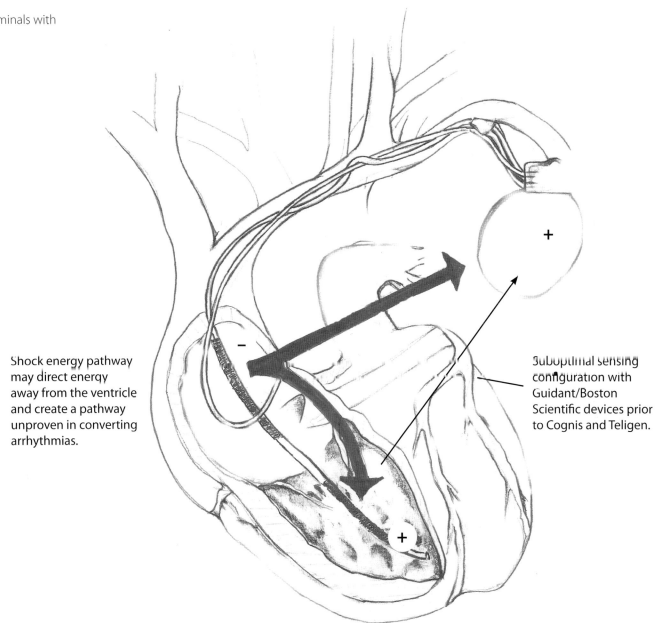

Shock energy pathway
may direct energy
away from the ventricle
and create a pathway
unproven in converting
arrhythmias.

Suboptimal sensing
configuration with
Guidant/Boston
Scientific devices prior
to Cognis and Teligen.

Figure 4.M.3

Medtronic device HV Pins reversed. May manifest as failed DFTs at implant. Notice the dissimilar pattern on Can to RV Ring and Can to RV Coil.

Panel A: Can to RV Ring

Panel B: Can to RV Coil

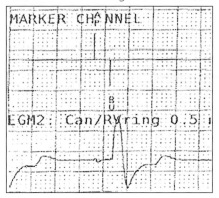
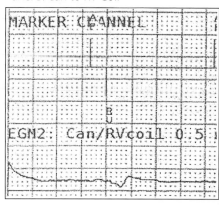

Figure 4.M.4

Medtronic device HV Pins connected correctly. Adequate DFTs. Consistent pattern on EGMs Can to RV Ring and Can to RV Coil.

Panel A: Can to RV Ring

Panel B: Can to RV Coil

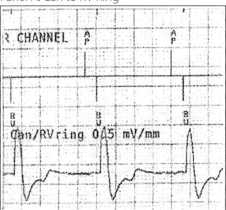
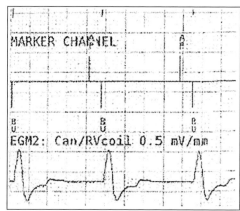

Figure 4.M.5

Guidant devices prior to Cognis/Teligen family HV Pins reversed. The Shock EGM utilizes data from the proximal and distal coils and the can. This may present with: large P waves in SR, Noise on RV and Shock EGM, reproducible with isometrics and failed DFT at implant.

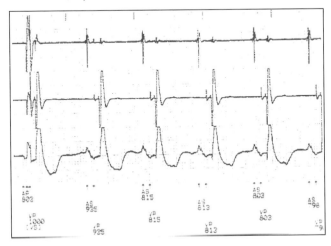

Figure 4.M.6

Boston Scientific device Teligen Device with HV Pins reversed. Shock EGM stored utilizing Can to Distal Coil. Manifests as large P wave on Shock EGM in SR. P wave and R wave similar in size. May manifest as failed DFTs at implant.

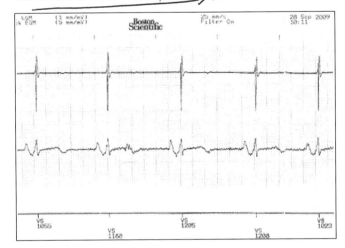

Figure 4.M.7

Boston Scientific Cognis device with HV Pins connected correctly.

Large artifact on Shock EGM consistent with RV activity. No atrial activity on Shock EGM. Adequate DFTs.

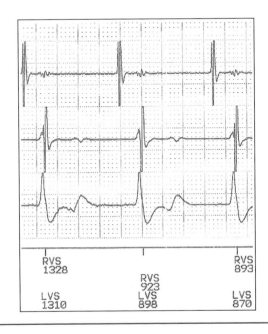

Reference

1. Issa Z. Inadvertent transposition of defibrillator coil terminal pins causing inappropriate ICD therapies. *J Cardiovasc Electrophysiol.* 2008;22:71-74.

2. Pai RK, Abedin M, Rawling DA. Inappropriate ICD shocks for inappropriate reasons. *Indian Pacing Electrophysiol J.* 2008;8:69-71.

3. Chawla P, Hanon S, Lam P, Schweitzer P. An uncommon cause of myopotentials leading to inappropriate ICD therapy. *Pacing Clin Electrophysiol.* 2009;32:1584-1586.

4. Jeevanantham V, Levine E, Budzikowski AS, Shah AH, Daubert JP. Defibrillation coil reversal: a rare cause of abnormal noise and inappropriate shocks. *Pacing Clin Electrophysiol.* 2008;31:375-377.

5. Kowalski M, Ellenbogen KA, Wood MA, Friedman P. Implantable cardiac defibrillators lead failure or myopotential oversensing? An approach to the diagnosis of noise on lead electrograms. *Europace.* 2008,10:914-917.

6. Weretka S, Michaelsen J, Becker R, et al. Ventricular oversensing: a study of 101 patients implanted with dual chamber defibrillators and two different lead systems. *Pacing Clin Electrophysiol.* 2003;26:65-70.

Appendix A

Spoiler alert! Because the case titles are by diagnosis, they may suggest an answer to the case question. Therefore they are presented as an appendix, rather than as a table of contents.

Appendix B